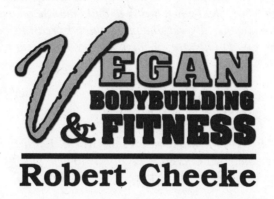

Robert Cheeke

"Before I found VeganBodybuilding.com, I was working my way down from an obese weight and wanted to build a decent physique once I lost my weight. I came to the forum section of Robert's website and found so much information and support there. Robert had some meal plans posted which I used to give myself an idea of what to eat when trying to build muscle on a vegan diet. The atmosphere there is generally very helpful, which I credit Robert for. He is a dynamic speaker, great motivator, positive person, and great human being."

Jacob Park
Writer, Personal Trainer
Chicago, IL

"Even though I live on the other side of the world, I still find myself being inspired and motivated by Robert and his ability to bring the best out of everyone he speaks to, which is a true testament of his character."

Joel Kirkilis
Vegan bodybuilder and Power lifter
Melbourne, Australia

"Not only has Robert been successful as a bodybuilder, but he has reached this point without putting any toxins in his body: no steroids, no drugs or alcohol, not even any meat or dairy products. He is very influential because he leads by example and doesn't compromise when it comes to what he stands for."

Dylan Kasprzyk
Comedian, Radio Sales Representative, Long-time Friend
Portland, OR

"Robert is all about a positive attitude and getting the most out of it, and I believe that if most people would act the same, there would be a much better understanding between all human beings."

Eran Blecher
Friend
Israel

"Robert's deep knowledge of the human body, vegan nutrition and training protocols is unmatched. Not only does Robert show that a peak-performer can get everything they need from a plant-based diet, he proves that this diet may be the best single change athletes can make for themselves. Anyone who wants to look and feel better will love this book!"

Alexandra Jamieson, CHHC, AADP
Vegan Nutrition Expert and Author of *Living Vegan for Dummies*
New York, NY

"As a friend who has known Robert since elementary school, I can attest to Robert's consistent ability over the years to motivate and inspire others through his actions. He has been, and is still known for his legendary enthusiasm and his ability to set goals and achieve them—often with stunning success. As long as I have known him, he has always been an enthusiastic, energizing, and inspiring figure. Seeing Robert over the past ten years accomplish so much in terms of becoming a successful businessman and one of the most recognizable vegan icons on the planet has been remarkable."

Jordan Baskerville
Long-time friend, Robert's first training partner
Corvallis, OR

"Robert doesn't just lift weights; he lifts up the entire vegan athletic culture with his website as an inspirational resource. He presses viewers to reach their personal best in this positive community built around health and fitness. Robert fosters a society where support to reach goals is given, sharing of ideas enhances vegan culture, and networking of common interests is realized. Robert personally 'spots' this community to achieve more than they could have on their own."

Mary Stella Stabinsky
Crossfit Trainer/ Veganbodybuilding.com member
Wilkes-Barre, PA

"Through his unmatched enthusiasm, contagious positivity, motivational message, and always with a little help from some well-earned biceps, Robert Cheeke is the perfect exemplification that a healthy lifestyle is overflowing with rewards."

Julie Morris
Writer, Graphic Designer, Vegan Chef
www.JulieMorris.net
Los Angeles, CA

"There is no one more qualified to write about being a vegan and a successful athlete. Robert lives it every day."

Nick Martin
Software developer, Entrepreneur, Author
Corvallis, OR

"Robert Cheeke is one heck of a vegan bodybuilder! I joined his website veganbodybuilding.com in late 2007. All I can say is wow! It totally changed my life."

Hayley Suska
Friend, ISCA certified personal trainer, writer
Orlando, FL

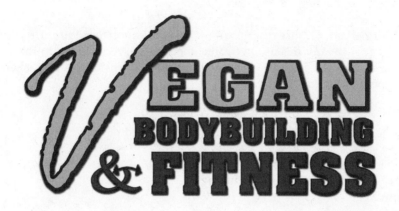

by Robert Cheeke

Healthy Living Publications
Summertown, Tennessee

Front cover photos:
Left- by Brian Van Peski
Center- by George Wong
Right- by Randall Perez - Randallperez.com

www.robertcheeke.com
www.veganbodybuilding.com

Healthy Living Publications
an imprint of Book Publishing Company
415 Farm Road
PO Box 99
Summertown, TN 38483
1-888-260-8458
www.bookpubco.com

ISBN: 978-0-9843916-0-8

Printed in Canada

Book Publishing Company is a member of Green Press Initiative. We chose to print this title on paper with 100% postconsumer recycled content, processed without chlorine, which saved the following natural resources:

- 91 trees
- 2,521 pounds of solid waste
- 41,524 gallons of water
- 8,622 pounds of greenhouse gases
- 29 million BTU of energy

green
press
INITIATIVE

For more information about Green Press Initiative visit www.greenpressinitiative.org. Environmental impact estimates were made using the Environmental Defense Fund Paper Calculator. For more information visit www.papercalculator.org.

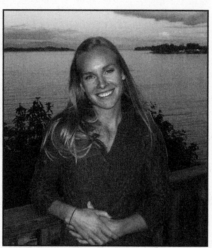

photo by Robert Cheeke

Edited by Julia Abbott, CPA
Author of the Lemon Letter Wellness Blog
and competitive runner based in Portland, Oregon
www.lemonletter.blogspot.com

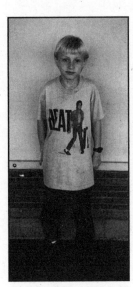

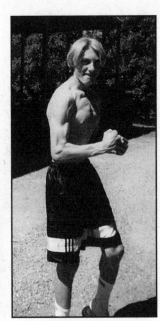

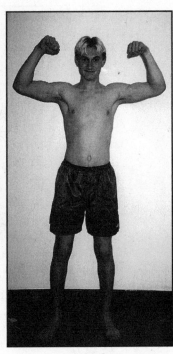

Age 10

Age 16
(photo by Clarke Cheeke)

Age 20

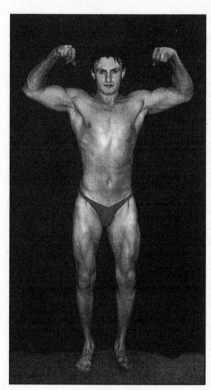

Age 23
(photo by Eric Brown)

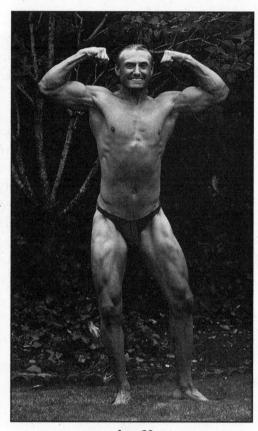

Age 29
(photo by Randall Perez)
RandallPerez.com

Disclaimer

The contents in this book have not been approved by the FDA or any other governing body concerning the nutrition and fitness advice and suggestions provided. They are the recommendations of vegan bodybuilder Robert Cheeke based on his experiences and are to be used as guidelines and models, not to be followed exactly.

Do not attempt to follow the nutrition or exercise suggestions without first consulting your physician. Robert Cheeke, the editors, publishers, printers, and others involved in this publication release themselves from any liability involving injury or loss as a result of applying the recommendations within this book.

Robert Cheeke is not a certified expert in nutrition or exercise and does not claim to be. In this book he simply shares his experiences learned over the past 14 years as a successful vegan athlete.

Above all, use reason and common sense, and be healthy and happy!

Table of Contents

Dedication

This book is dedicated to the www.veganbodybuilding.com members and online vegan athlete forum community. Thank you all for your generous support over the past eight years! You are a wonderful group of people, and I am thrilled to have you in my life. Thank you for all that you are and for all that you do. You are the best!

I also dedicate this book to the billions of lives lost because of our irresponsible mistreatment of animals. With this book and many more to come, I aim to give hope to a brighter future for all of us.

Finally, I dedicate this book to those of you who believed in me when nobody else would. I wasn't expected to succeed the way I have, but I believed I would and so did you. You know who you are, and I am forever grateful for your unconditional support.

Make the best of this one life you have and enjoy every day of it.

Robert at the Ching Farm Animal Sanctuary (photo by Crystal Hammer)

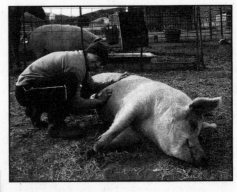

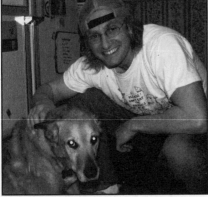

Robert with Razor, one of the best dogs ever (photo by Mary Ann Tarr)

Acknowledgements

It is no secret that I enjoy recognizing the people in my life who have supported me, influenced me in inspirational fashion, or have otherwise contributed to my life in positive ways. With every book I write, I love to take the opportunity right up front to acknowledge a special group of people and thank them for the role they have played in my life.

There are some people who deserve to be acknowledged because of the role models they have been for me and because they have inspired me down a similar path of success. Some are unlikely heroes of mine who have become my mentors, and others are great friends who seem to stand by me no matter what outlandish visions for my future I share with them.

I have a complete list of acknowledgements on the book website www.veganbodybuildingbook.com, but up front I wanted to thank the following people for their support of this specific project:

Julia Abbott, Michael Arnesen, Gary Asher, Jordan Baskerville, Brendan Brazier, Tracy Brown, Charles Chang, Edna Cheeke, Peter Cheeke, Tanya Cheeke, Joseph Connelly, Jody Conners, Kevin Gianni, Sam Harris, Randall Perez, Ravi Raman, Brian Van Peski, and Richard Watts.

I want to thank everyone else who has supported this book and Vegan Bodybuilding & Fitness over the years, as well as all of the people who provided a testimonial for me to be included in this book. Many thanks to all of you! Thank you to those who support my company, my personal brand, and all of my other dreams, visions, and other projects too. It is all greatly appreciated!

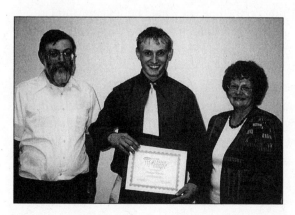

Robert with mother Edna and father Peter at UCMT graduation in 2000.

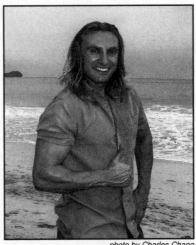

photo by Charles Chang

About the Author

Allow me to tell you a little bit about myself. I'm your new best friend because I'm the guy who's going to help you achieve the dreams even you thought were out of reach. I'll be there to support you even when times are tough, so you're going to want to get to know me a little better. Above all else, I'm a nice guy. That is how I prefer to be recognized first, before anything else—not as an author, a motivational speaker, a vegan bodybuilder, or a leader, but first and foremost, just a really nice guy. After all, nice guys finish first, right? If you meet someone who is nicer than I, please let me know and I'll alter my behavior to take the title back. It is *that* important to me. I am authentic down to the core, and I care immensely about meaningful things in my life. I put everything on the line for what I believe in, and I allow myself to be completely transparent. Transparency is a very important aspect of my life; it is a key factor in how others get to know who I really am and what I'm all about.

I grew up on a farm in the small college town of Corvallis, Oregon with my parents, my older sister, and two younger brothers. I enjoyed childhood and spent a lot of time playing with my siblings and the farm animals we had on the 20-acre property. I even recall having a pet housefly, and I was compassionate towards all beings way back then. I was careful not to step on ants, had a soft spot for lonely or injured animals, and had the same character traits then that I have now with regard to being considerate and respectful toward everything around me. Being surrounded by the playfulness and innocence of farm animals proved to be an important factor of my childhood. Many of the animals on our farm had first names just like me, and it was at a young age I first recognized a significant connection between humans and animals that was deeper than just servant and master.

For as long as I can remember, I've been a dreamer, visualizing great achievements and being determined to reach high levels of success. I was convinced that I could discover what I was naturally good at, learn to enjoy it, and make a living out of it. Subsequently, I was also convinced that I could make a success out of something I was only satisfactory at but enjoyed immensely, if only I dedicated the time to learn to do it better. Following my heart has been the true key to my success in life. I tested my theory of having fun while succeeding at what I really loved to do, and it worked in nearly every area of interest. I have journal entries from when I was a teenager outlining some of the goals for my life that ten years later I am achieving. It is at these times I feel most content and most fulfilled knowing I did what most don't think they will ever be able to do—actually live out a childhood dream.

My background is multifaceted and includes pursuits in health and fitness, world travel, communication, public speaking, business management, motivational lectures, leadership, writing, massage therapy, competitive bodybuilding, working with children, and event organizing. In whatever activity I am involved, lifting others up around me has always been a primary goal. When I learned how to do it effectively, my impact on my community was more significant than I could have imagined. Dedicating my life to inspiring and lifting up others has been one of the most rewarding pursuits I have ever undertaken. Inspiration is something I hope to instill in many people throughout my life. I live a life of service to the causes I care most about.

Currently, I live in Portland, Oregon, and I love it here. That's how it should be. If you don't love where you live, you should move or learn to love where you are. Portland has been great for me to grow as a person and develop as a business person. Based on my lifestyle, it has been the ideal place to network and increase my own reputation in the health, fitness, and personal development communities. I also have family and friends in and around Portland, which further establishes this great city as "home" for me.

I follow a plant-based diet and encourage others to do the same for optimal health and vitality, to live compassionately, and to leave less of a footprint on our Earth when we leave. I've been following a pure plant-based diet since 1996 and will continue with this lifestyle forever. This lifestyle forever changed my life for the better, and that is something I will never forget. It has been through my vegan diet (no animal products) and lifestyle that I have built my reputation as one of the most influential vegan athletes on the planet.

I am the founder and President of my own company (Vegan Bodybuilding & Fitness–established in 2002) and the Director and Producer of the Award-Winning Documentary *Vegan Fitness Built Naturally (2005)* and Co-Director and Co-Producer of the documentary *Vegan Brothers in Iron* (scheduled to be released in 2010). I am the author of *Take Action and Make it Happen – Bringing Out the Best in You* and *Your Personal Best*, books that were written in 2008 and scheduled to be released in 2010 and 2011. I am the producer of *The Robert Cheeke Show* and determined to create many more innovative programs. I am a competitive bodybuilder, motivational speaker, author, actor, fitness model, event organizer, and friend to a lot of people all over the world. I'm also honorary uncle to more kids than I can keep up with, and it's great!

At the time of this writing, I am 29 years old, single, and can often be found traveling around North America speaking at various health, wellness, vegetarian, personal development, and fitness festivals. Look for the blond guy with a big smile, muscles, and lots of enthusiasm. If that guy is flexing for the camera, dancing to hip hop music, or playing with a group of kids, it's most likely me. Come up to me and say hi. I love meeting new people. You will also likely find me on a motivational speaking tour because that has been my new focus—speaking to Universities and other groups all over the United States. I started writing this book when I was 28 years old, and I am determined to become a best-selling author by age 30. Thank you for supporting my efforts to make this happen. I will be on a massive book tour starting in February 2010, and I would love to come to your town! Email me at robert@veganbodybuilding.com, and let's figure out a way to add your city to my book tour schedule.

My whole theme in life is to be happy, to be nice to others, and to be motivated to positively change the world in whatever way suits me. I'm determined, dedicated, and persistent. I care about cause and effect and the outcomes of actions, and I am driven to inspire and motivate others. My vision is to be right more than wrong, happy more than sad, nice more than mean, caring more than apathetic, and to live without limits. I have a great family and wonderful friends. I have had some incredible role models in my life who have impacted me in immeasurable ways and simultaneously built my character to be strong and steadfast becoming a leader in my communities.

I have an uplifting, encouraging, and inspiring story to share with as many people as I can. Thank you for taking the time to read my book. It is my sincere desire that it encourages you to be the best at something important in your life. Thank you for giving me the opportunity to inspire you. I wish you all the best along your journey. I am always here to support you. Find me on www.veganbodybuilding.com and contact me anytime. Connect with me on social media websites like Facebook, Twitter, and YouTube. Just search my name and I'll be there. All the best!

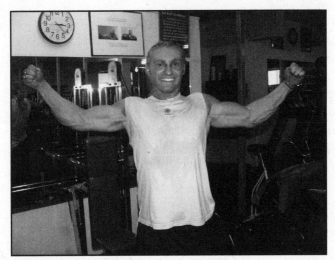

Training at Loprinzi's Gym, Portland, Oregon.
(photo by Giacomo Marchese)

Introduction

The idea of vegan bodybuilding has long been perceived as an oxymoron until now. In an industry riddled with animal-derived body-enhancing supplements, a new wave of bodybuilding is emerging. For the past ten years I have been at the forefront, pioneering a different way to fuel and nourish bodybuilders while nourishing the planet at the same time.

This book is well overdue, and I am pleased to finally bring it to life and have it available to an audience that has been craving its completion for years. This complete guide to proper training and plant-based nutrition for athletes has been a decade in the making, following my career as a vegan bodybuilder over the past ten years. Of the nearly seven billion people on the planet, my name has been synonymous with vegan bodybuilding more than any other name in history. My name, my face, and my physique have been the most recognized in this industry throughout the world, and that makes it very fitting for me to deliver this book in a very unique way that is sure to motivate and inspire anyone.

I come from the unlikely background of being a skinny farm boy who grew up eating meat and selling animals at 4-H auctions to be slaughtered for food. I was born into a family who has had farming in its history for generations, and I'm the son of farmers who both worked in a university Animal

Science department. But the choices I have made and the passion that has supported them enable me to stand out in the world of vegan bodybuilding.

Many asked why I hadn't written this book sooner. The truth is that I started a book about vegan health and athletics back in 2003 and continued working on it again 2005. My life took a turn in a new direction in the middle of that year when I directed and produced the documentary *Vegan Fitness Built Naturally*. Immediately, as a result of that documentary, I was hired by Sequel Naturals to work for Vega. I spent half the year traveling around the country to work at consumer wellness shows and festivals and give talks. Writing this book took a back seat while inspiring as many people as possible through in-person interaction and training in the gym became my top priorities. When I finally returned to the project, I sat down in front of the computer, started over on page one, and wrote over 100 pages in the first four days. With a decade of experience as a vegan bodybuilder, everything about this book became not only easy to write about but also extremely rewarding and fulfilling.

Because of the unique approach I took to incorporate some of my personal development and success strategies, this book will be the most comprehensive guide to building your body on a plant-based diet and an ever-present source of motivation. This book is designed to answer any question about vegan bodybuilding you could possibly have. The content addresses more than what to eat, how to train, and what supplements to take as a vegan bodybuilder; it includes far more than inspirational photos of vegan bodybuilders. The book contains 15 chapters of the most important components of successful bodybuilding on a plant-based diet: how to get sponsored by companies and make a career out of your bodybuilding hobby; ways to stay motivated and find meaning in your actions; lists of do's and don'ts when it comes to the sport of bodybuilding; lists of products, services, and equipment that are vegan; meal programs and training programs; and how to turn your vegan bodybuilding lifestyle into extremely effective forms of activism and outreach.

Even more than vegan bodybuilding and fitness, this book is about the pursuit of excellence—making the most out of your life and contributing to the world in ways that you never imagined. It is about inspiring you to do amazing things while causing the least amount of harm and doing the most amount of good. You can't delegate passion, it has to come from within, but you can inspire passion in others by leading by positive example.

I chose to specifically include brand names of products that I use or recommend. I did not receive any compensation for my recommendations from any company. I am only sharing the truth as I know it from my direct experience. I share a variety of products in multiple categories of nutrition because each person responds uniquely to each product. I will list brands of equipment and supplies, as well as my favorite places to train and eat by name and location along with menu recommendations. This will be an excellent overall resource for motivation, inspiration, vegan living, bodybuilding, and bringing out the best in you.

There are some repetitive themes throughout this book which is intentional by design. Philosopher Daniel Dennett, Professor at Tufts University, said in a Technology, Entertainment, and Design (TED) talk in 2008, "Every time you read it or say it you make another copy in your brain." Professor Dennett is explaining that repetition helps with retention. Therefore, the reader benefits with sustained knowledge rather than temporary memorization.

Thank you for taking the time to care enough to support me, my ambitions for the world, and the vegan cause. Thank you for supporting the concept of Vegan Bodybuilding & Fitness, for picking this book up, for reading it cover to cover, for sharing it with friends, and for providing me feedback about how I can make it better.

I wish you all the best on your journey to great strength, great health, great fulfillment, and great contribution. Welcome to the world of Vegan Bodybuilding & Fitness. Take your ticket…it's show time! Whatever it is that moves you, whatever it is that drives you, go after it and make it happen today.

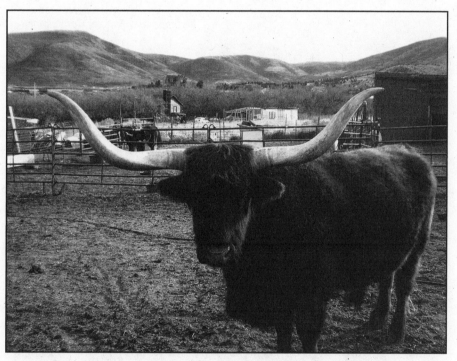

One of the many rescued animals Robert is committed to supporting
(photo by Robert Cheeke)

"Through his award-winning bodybuilding career and his promotion of veganism, Robert Cheeke has inspired and motivated not only athletes around the world but also everyday people to adopt a vegan lifestyle. His integrity and his commitment to the plight of animal rights and environmentalism truly reflect a consciousness in action and global responsibility, thus leading to a positive impact on and contribution to society."

John Pierre
Nutrition and Fitness Consultant
Chicago, IL

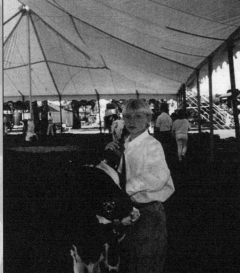

Showing a dairy calf in 4-H

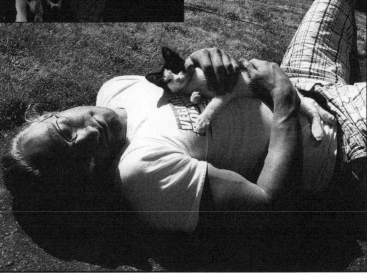

(photo by Natasha West)

Chapter 1

Why Vegan?

"Do we, as humans, having an ability to reason and to communicate abstract ideas verbally and in writing, and to form ethical and moral judgments using the accumulated knowledge of the ages, have the right to take the lives of other sentient organisms, particularly when we are not forced to do so by hunger or dietary need, but rather do so for the somewhat frivolous reason that we like the taste of meat? In essence, should we know better?"

Peter Cheeke, PhD
Contemporary Issues in Animal Agriculture, 2004

If we're going to have a "Vegan" Bodybuilding book we may as well start right from the very beginning: Why vegan in the first place? What does it mean, and why would we want to incorporate it into a bodybuilding program or into our lives? Furthermore, how can we best represent and promote the vegan cause?

Vegan, by definition means: "a vegetarian who eats plant products only, especially one who uses no products derived from animals, as fur or leather," according to www.freedictionary.com. A vegan is basically someone who abstains from consuming or using any animal products, animal by-products, and products that are tested on animals. Each individual may have their own political agenda that adds another component to their description or definition of veganism; but in general, for common explanations, vegans do not eat or use anything that comes from an animal, and they do not contribute to animal cruelty or suffering. In fact, not only do vegans not contribute to animal suffering, they work hard to eradicate animal suffering through diet, lifestyle, activism, and outreach.

From a social, environmental, ethical, and health standpoint, adopting a vegan lifestyle is a practical and smart choice for anyone. First of all, causing harm to others, including animals, is not very nice and completely unnecessary. The environment suffers from the methane emitted from livestock; the air and water are deteriorated by animal waste from factory farms; and consumption of animal products is directly linked to heart disease and obesity. A vegan lifestyle solves all these problems. If you stop for a moment to consider it, consumption of one hamburger impacts much more than one's digestion. The vegan lifestyle is a compassionate way to live that supports life, supports fairness and equality, and promotes freedom.

My decision to switch from an animal-based diet to a plant-based diet came about through the inspiration, leadership, and influence of my older sister Tanya. At a young age she decided to become a vegan while we were growing up on a farm. She was convinced that living a vegan lifestyle was most in line with her personal feelings toward animals as friends rather than food. She was outspoken among our family and at Corvallis High School, which we attended in the mid 1990's. She was so outspoken about the abuse animals endure as a result of human behavior that she organized an Animal Rights Week at our school. For no other reason than respect for Tanya, I decided that I would participate in the animal rights week. It began on December 8, 1995, and that was the beginning of a new life for me. I told my friends David Foster and Jordan Baskerville that I would no longer be going out to lunch with them everyday at fast food restaurants and sandwich shops. I didn't know it at the time, but that decision I made December 8, 1995 brought me to where I am today. I also didn't know that 14 years later David would be vegan and Jordan would be a near vegetarian flirting with the idea of veganism and one of my biggest supporters of my vegan bodybuilding

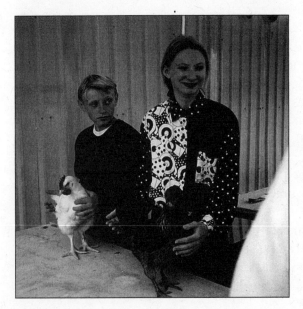

Robert with older sister Tanya showing chickens in 4-H at the county fair

career. The three of us remain great friends today, and I am so thankful to have them in my life.

During the Animal Rights Week, I attended events all week long. I listened to presenters, read literature, and watched videos of animal testing and factory farming. The information I learned and the images I saw were enough to get me to change my entire lifestyle—adopt a vegetarian diet immediately and a full vegan lifestyle months later. In fact, two years later, I was organizing the Animal Rights Week at Corvallis High School as a senior. Little did I know that it was the beginning of the activism and outreach and event organizing that I continue to do today on much larger scales to greater audiences.

My vegan lifestyle wasn't perfect, however. I had arguments with friends, got kicked out of class for being outspoken about political issues related to animal rights, and spent a couple of years frustrated and angry towards society—something I see in many activists today. I was angry at my family and angry at my friends. I said some things to some important people in my life that I regret. I can't change the past, but I can apologize to the people I was mean to, including my own family members. I recall telling my dad that he was a bad father for raising us to eat meat. I remember burning money because I thought it was worthless if it was going to be used to buy animal products. While those are actions and concepts I believed in then, they weren't very nice things. They didn't make a difference, and I apologize for the behavior that was counter-productive to the movement and mean to the people in my life who were trying to understand my new passion and interests as a renegade teenager.

Things have changed a lot since then, and I have learned to be happy because I'm vegan rather than sad or angry because others are not. I have learned how to interact and communicate with people effectively, have intellectual conversations, and speak in terms that are not condescending or rude or in ways that will turn people off from me or my messages. I have also learned how to think about the big picture—about what really matters most and how my actions are impacting the lives of those I'm trying to save. I changed a lot of my behavior, and as a result, I have been much more effective in promoting the message of veganism in a positive way. Long gone are the days of an angry and frustrated vegan bodybuilder.

So what does bodybuilding and fitness have to do with the vegan cause? Being physically fit is a way to draw positive attention to the vegan movement. Being exceptional illustrates to others that there is more to being vegan than is readily apparent; it breaks through predispositions and biased thinking. It destroys the common programming of what proper diet and exercise are. It piques curiosity, welcomes a closer look, and incites discussion and inquiry from those outside the movement. At this point, the positive, fit vegan should be equipped to engage the curious in logical conversation that highlights the immense good the vegan movement strives to create in the world. The positive, fit vegan should inspire and motivate impactful change in every personal encounter.

Robert's Recap on Why Vegan

As I've said all along, living a cruelty-free lifestyle is the nice thing to do and if that was our best argument for veganism, it would be good enough for me. By nature, as humans we want to be nice to others. This is seen in all facets of our behavior. We are a caring and nurturing species who enjoys doing good things and enjoys the fulfillment we get from doing nice things for others. Avoiding the use of animal products and animal by-products and standing up for something meaningful is a great way to approach life. This lifestyle has many benefits. By following a plant-based diet you will likely have lower cholesterol levels and likely have increased energy because that is what plant-based foods provide naturally. Living a vegan lifestyle can provide a vast array of unique opportunities for you to thrive in all areas of life. Think about what it means to believe in something and to make a difference in the world from a practical, reasonable, sensible, and logical standpoint. Consider living a vegan lifestyle and go vegan today!

Robert's Top 10 Reasons to Go Vegan!

1. It is the nice thing to do. Harming animals is not very nice and is in fact very mean and cruel.

2. Eating plants rather than animals is a more long-term, sustainable solution for our planet.

3. A plant-based diet is natural: If children had to witness the slaughter of animals, they would likely never want to be part of anything related to animal cruelty. Our most honest and sincere citizens can often tell what is right and what is wrong, and we can learn from them.

4. Going vegan enables you to become part of a new community of other like-minded people determined to impact the world in positive ways. It's always fun to join a new group of people, make new friends, and be part of something productive.

5. In most cases animals can't defend themselves against the human's bullying ways, be it related to factory farming or animal testing or

other areas of mistreatment. Going vegan and standing up for animals gives them hope and gives them a chance to live a free life like humans get to live.

6. You will likely not be one of the 200 million people in the United States who are suffering from diet-related illnesses (obesity, high cholesterol, heart problems, the clogging of arteries, etc.) if you follow a plant-based whole food diet.

7. You will have more meaning in your life knowing you're making a difference in the lives of many animals simply by not killing them or having someone else kill them for you.

8. If you had to kill an animal with your bare hands each and every time you wanted to eat meat, you probably couldn't do it; therefore you probably shouldn't eat it.

9. Becoming vegan makes you stand out and break away from the norm. It makes you become more marketable as an athlete, more unique as an individual, and makes you more well rounded as it adds another interesting component to your lifestyle.

10. A diet higher in carbohydrates provides more energy, and plant-based whole foods are packed full of carbohydrates, vitamins, minerals, amino acids, fatty acids, protein and essential fats.

"Health and Fitness have always been a big part of my life, and when I became vegan this was no different. As I embraced my new lifestyle I began to feel a little alienated from the main stream bodybuilding community and began to wonder if it was even possible to stay strong and build muscle on a vegan diet. When I discovered Robert's Vegan Bodybuilding and Fitness website and ultimately met Robert in person, it changed the way I looked at veganism and gave me a new found belief in the vegan way of life. Since then, Robert has continued to motivate me in my training and helped me to represent veganism in a healthy and positive way. His dedication to the cause and the promotion of veganism has brought together a group of inspirational and awe-inspiring people and helped to build a strong vegan bodybuilding community."

Chris Rowe
Rugby Player
Sydney, Australia

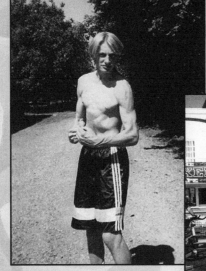

Robert at age 16
(photo by Clarke Cheeke)

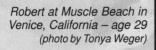

Robert at Muscle Beach in
Venice, California – age 29
(photo by Tonya Weger)

Chapter 2

Beginning Bodybuilding –
How to get started in bodybuilding
and achieve results

"Vegan bodybuilding is about fueling your body with a vast array of natural, healthy foods, combined with resistance weight training and exercise, providing your body with the appropriate tools to build your physique and achieve your fitness goals."

Robert Cheeke, Author

I'm often asked how it all started for me—how I got into bodybuilding in the first place. Allow me to take you down memory lane to paint a picture of what mattered to me as a young boy driven and determined to be the person I grew up to be. This is my story. This is where it all began, and this is what means so much to me. My hope is that it inspires a dream in you, new or long forgotten, fitness-related or not.

One of my oldest memories is dressing up for Halloween as a kindergarten He-Man—the muscle-bound, fictional cartoon character with a fake tan and long blond hair who spreads positive messages to his audience. At five years of age I believed that if I worked hard enough, it really would happen. And it did. I worked so hard, every day from that day on, never losing sight of my goal. Approximately 25 years later—with my long blond hair, muscles, and fake tan—I became my childhood hero, sharing positive messages with people all over the world.

As far back as I can remember, I flexed my tiny muscles in front of a mirror every single day—from when I was a kid, through high school, and into my 20's. It was a form of affirmation supporting my childhood dream I had as a kindergartner. Like clockwork, I wouldn't miss a day and attributed my muscle definition to the fact that I flexed my biceps for at least a moment every single day. I continue this daily flexing ritual today at nearly 30 years of age. This seemingly insignificant practice helped support my earliest ambi-

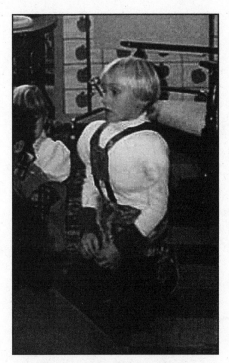

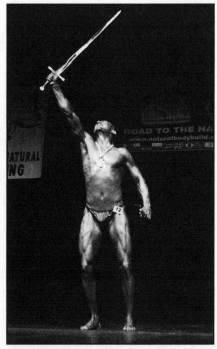

Robert at age 5 dressed up as He-Man in Kindergarten

Robert winning the 2009 INBA Northwestern USA Natural Bodybuilding Championships becoming a real life He-Man, complete with victory sword (photo by Shauna Shelton)

tions and turn them into reality. How many five-year-olds know who and what they want to be when they grow up and actually have the ability to follow their dreams and follow each essential step throughout their lives to make it happen without wavering or losing sight of their childhood dream? Not many. That ritual of flexing everyday was also the beginning of the theme that proved to play the most important role in my life thereafter: the rule of consistency. Nobody loves consecutive streaks more than I do; my focus on consistency in action has made me successful in all areas of life I have applied it. I once completed a predetermined number of push-ups and sit-ups everyday for 839 consecutive days because I knew that kind of dedication to consistency would pay off in other areas of life as well as define my arms, chest, and shoulders.

In addition to wanting to be like He-Man, I wanted to be a professional wrestler like Hulk Hogan. He was another blond haired, fake tanned muscle guy who was a positive role model, promoting positive messages and leading by example. I got involved in organized wrestling for two years before the age of ten. I lifted weights for the first time at age 14 when I won a trial membership at Downing's Gym in Corvallis, OR. With the vision of being like He-Man and Hulk Hogan, I set out to be the best at everything from academics to athletics. I was above average at everything because of that attitude.

I had a problem though. I was very small. To put it into perspective, I was the shortest boy in my 4th grade class. Though I was active and excelled on the athletic field, track, and court, in the 8th grade I was between 4'11" & 5'1" in height and weighed 89 ¼ pounds. I was small. In fact, I was really small for my age. But I was determined to get bigger and stronger. I obviously had a long road ahead because of my size and because of the size of my future goals to be a person of large size and stature. I never really felt like giving up, I just knew it would take some time for me to put on muscle and get bigger and stronger. I enjoyed the challenge and always thought about the future and had a very clear understanding of where I was headed.

I was a late bloomer and entered puberty later than others, but over time my physique did change. At age 15, when I became a vegetarian, I weighed approximately 120 pounds. The following year as a vegan and a junior in high school, I wrestled at 133 pounds; I graduated high school at the bodyweight of about 150 pounds. I was starting to grow and gain muscle, but I was far from being a bodybuilder or resembling He-Man or any other fit fictional character known for their outstanding, carefully drawn, and artistically sculpted physique. I lifted weights throughout high school while on sports teams and in weight training class. I loved to write and to exercise, so I spent my summers exercising and recording my training sessions in journals. I ran, cycled, performed push-ups and sit-ups, lifted weights, and played sports including basketball and soccer.

Year by year I moved closer to bulking up. I had my younger brother Clarke take photos of me flexing as a high school student. I am so glad I did

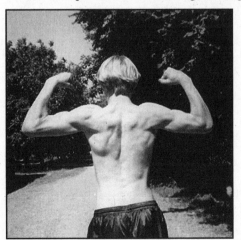

because I have those photos of a 16-year-old newly vegan kid with dreams of becoming bigger to look back on. Even though I was pretty small, I was always lean and had lots of visible veins and muscle definition. I always thought it was a result of my daily ritual of flexing in front of the mirror for a few

Robert, age 16
(photo by Clarke Cheeke)

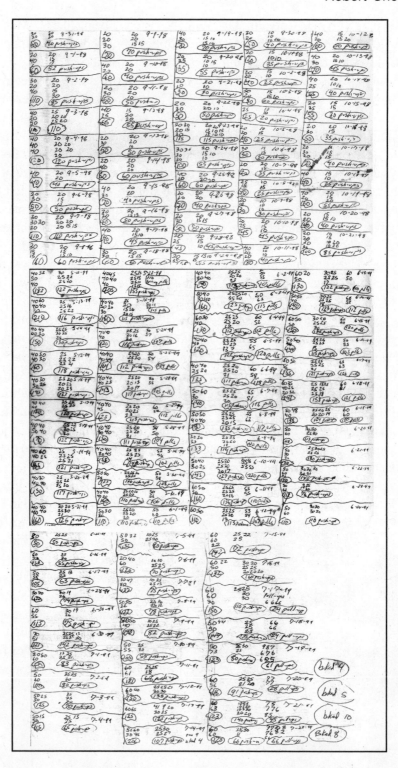

seconds. I thought as long as I did that a couple of times daily like brushing my teeth, my muscles would grow in bulk and definition. I enjoyed this journey so much that my high school senior yearbook portrait is a photo of me with my shirt off flexing my 140-pound vegan muscle physique uniquely placed among portraits of my classmates wearing nice clothes in professionally posed portraits. I was so pleased with the muscle photos Clarke took while I worked toward becoming a professional wrestler, I showed them to my leadership teacher Jon Bullock who also shared a passion for professional wrestling. More than ten years later, Mr. Bullock and I are still in

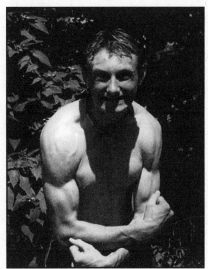

Robert's senior photo in the high school yearbook
(photo by Clarke Cheeke)

touch. His belief in my abilities to do great things helped me throughout my life as I worked ferociously to make dreams come true. He taught me to "Demand Excellence" and that is a standard I have held myself to over the past decade.

Bodybuilding didn't come as easy as I thought it would. The fact is, bodybuilding isn't easy, and it has to be done properly. Otherwise, it will be frustrating, unsuccessful, not enjoyable, and not worthwhile. Bodybuilding didn't come easily for me because I wasn't putting in the time necessary to create the changes in my body I hoped to see in a short amount of time. It is often assumed that all one has to do is lift weights and eat a bit more to suddenly be transformed to resemble the people who fill the pages of muscle magazines. I also thought that if I took supplements with images of bodybuilders on the bottle, I would automatically look like them over time whether I spent time in the gym or not. It just doesn't work that way and it can often take long periods of time before results are seen. The commitment can be enough to deter people from wanting to pursue the lifestyle any further. The specific reason bodybuilding didn't work for me at first was because I wasn't in the gym frequently enough to elicit physical change in my body. Additionally, I wasn't eating adequate amounts of food to support the times I was going to the gym. I was 19 years old; what do you think I was really doing? It wasn't training five or six days a week, but it was hanging out with my friends until 3AM, chasing after girls, sleeping in, going out dancing, and being involved in social activities. I never gave myself a fighting chance to adapt in the gym and build muscle. I was too busy doing what most teenagers do, and I wasn't as focused as I needed to be.

When I finally utilized the discipline and proper behaviors that bodybuilding requires, I began to see desired results. Furthermore, I began to understand how to adapt my training to affect changes in my body. Effective practice gave me the confidence to pursue bodybuilding further. I realized that consistency is one of the most important keys to success in any area of life.

While consistency counts for a major portion of the difference between success and failure, it still isn't everything. I write about some of my struggles with the initial stages of my bodybuilding career extensively because it was much more than a lack of consistency in the gym; it was a whole change in psychological approach that enabled me to succeed when most people fail. The lessons I learned from being observant and aware of my actions, my failures, and my successes proved to be some of the most valuable lessons I learned about my life. Now, I clearly understand how to create a detailed vision and see it all the way through to outstanding levels of success. I learned to be exceptional by observing my own life over the past 15 years and by truly understanding what made me fail and what made me succeed. I have created a formula for success that I follow in everything I do, including bodybuilding. That formula for success in anything is the premise of my personal development books and is the foundation which all of my projects are based upon. I simply learned how to care more than most, work harder than most, and use my talents and skills in innovative ways to ensure success in anything.

For thoroughness, I will summarize my formula for success as it is presented in my personal development books below.

Step 1:   Create a detailed vision for success based around something you're passionate about.

Step 2:   Embrace your vision with enthusiasm and be consistent with your efforts.

Step 3:   Allow adaptation to occur.

Step 4:   Improve as a result of your consistent and dedicated actions.

Step 5:   Succeed and share your success with others, inspiring others to be remarkable.

In all areas of life, I have found that if you discover something that you are truly passionate about and work hard at it consistently, then adaptation, improvement, and ultimately success follow. Once success is achieved, others are naturally inspired, which gives you confidence to succeed in other areas of life too. There are lots of specific components including action plans, support networks, timelines, and other key areas to give attention, but if you just follow those five simple steps without knowing any more of the details, you're bound to be highly successful and live a very fulfilling life.

When bodybuilding started to make sense to me and I was able to make progress and understand why I was making progress, my career as a bodybuilder really took off. I was merely lifting weights until I met up with my old childhood friend Jordan Baskerville, the same friend I knew at age five and the friend I stopped going to lunch with in high school when I became a vegan. We met in person back in Corvallis when I returned from spending a year in college in Salt Lake City, UT. I didn't know the names of bodybuilders or the names of poses, and I didn't know anything about the competitive aspect of the sport. I only knew how to lift weights, push myself incredibly hard, and watch my body grow, adapt, and improve. Jordan and I talked enthusiastically about our shared interest in bodybuilding. He invited me to his house and showed me a bunch of FLEX magazines blanketed with bodybuilding images. He told me about some of the bodybuilders and professed his interest in bodybuilding. I hadn't seen Jordan since high school graduation, and I was thrilled to see him and to know that he shared a passion of mine. We immediately became training partners, and that jump-started my career as a bodybuilder. For the first time I thought about the possibilities of competing rather than just lifting weights. Jordan and I trained together on and off for years, traveled to bodybuilding events together meeting celebrity professional bodybuilders, and had some incredible times. We helped each other grow and watched one another succeed.

When we first started training together, I told Jordan that I would be in muscle magazines and that I

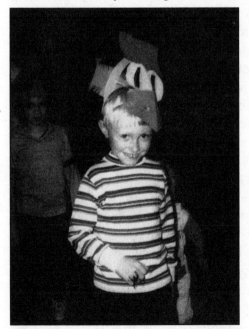

Robert with pre-school friend Jordan Baskerville who later introduced Robert to bodybuilding at age 20

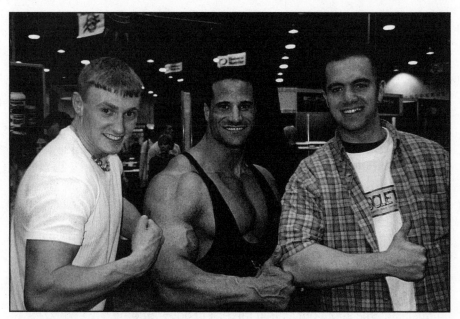

Robert, IFBB Pro Bodybuilder Mike Matarazzo and Jordan Baskerville

would fulfill some childhood dreams to make a name for myself and make a difference in the world. I honestly think he was quite skeptical about my ambitions, but he told me that he trusted I would indeed achieve what I set out to achieve. Years later, I appeared in millions of magazine issues from mainstream to obscure; I was featured in publications in many different countries all over the world. We had no idea at age 20 when we met by chance in Corvallis in the grocery store aisle that Jordan's influence on me would help me appear in FLEX Magazine three consecutive years and that I would be well on my way to being the most recognized vegan bodybuilder in the entire world. However, we both knew then that I had the potential to make it happen. Potential counts for a lot; but heart, desire, and will can take a dream from potential to possible.

Beginning Bodybuilding should be approached like beginning anything you want to be successful in. It starts with having a reason or meaning behind it, creating a detailed vision of what you want to achieve, and constructing and implementing a consistent program to ensure that you adapt, improve, and succeed. You also have to have a passion for it. If you don't have a desire that burns inside of you and inspires you completely, you won't be as motivated to do what you have to do day in and day out to achieve. Often, we are intimidated by the unknown; new or unfamiliar territory frightens us. If we realize that any new hobby or interest is like any new job or any new relationship, we can go into it with the same tools that we use to approach other areas of life that we care deeply about; we work hard to make sure everything is done at our very best. When we approach bodybuilding the same way, we create an atmosphere for success; we build a template for achievement and create the patterns that lead us to the destination we strive for. Bodybuilding can certainly be complicated, especially when talking about specific aspects of pre-contest preparation; but overall, it is as simple as anything else in life. It just takes effort, intent, and focus. Success can be found easier than you imagine.

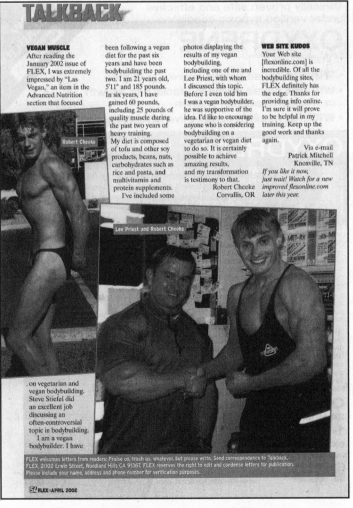

One of Robert's 3 features in FLEX Magazine

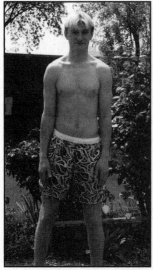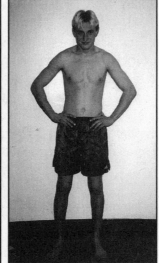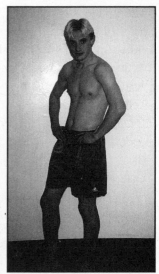

The day before beginning bodybuilding, summer 2000, weighing 157 pounds

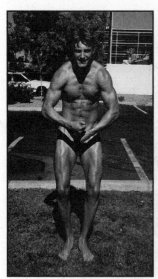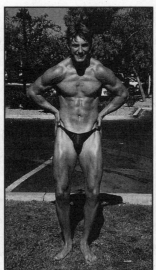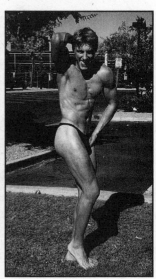

After one year of bodybuilding, spring 2001, weighing 185 pounds

The History of Vegan Bodybuilding & Fitness, the company I created

You know how and why I got into bodybuilding, and now I want to share with you the history of my company Vegan Bodybuilding & Fitness. I get the question all the time, "How did you get into Vegan Bodybuilding?" or "Tell me how you started your company."

Here is how the business of Vegan Bodybuilding & Fitness began:

As a vegan athlete for years, a vegan weight lifter by age 20, and a vegan bodybuilder by age 21, I decided it was time to start branding the concept to share my success with others. At the time, I didn't know any other vegan athletes, let alone other vegan bodybuilders, so it was my mission to pioneer the industry by starting a company and building a website to build a community around Vegan Bodybuilding & Fitness.

In 2002, I started my business Vegan Bodybuilding & Fitness in hope of becoming well known in the fitness industry and able to promote veganism on a world-wide level through my fitness lifestyle. My goal was to earn enough income through my company that I would not have to work a standard 9 to 5 job and so I could spend most of my time focusing on things I really enjoyed while making a difference. With the help from my friends Eric Brown and Tim Martin, I got my business and website off the ground in 2002. We launched our www.veganbodybuilder.com (now www.veganbodybuilding.com) website in 2003. Once off the ground, friends Khan Gorlewski and Richard Watts helped me maintain and grow my website over the years.

At first, the company didn't really have a lot to offer other than a website full of information, so the first business move I made was making t-shirts. While still on a cruise ship out in the Caribbean working as a massage therapist, I had a friend on board the ship draw up some initial sketches for logos. I had a handful of t-shirts printed in Florida, and they are the very first clothing items we ever made. When I got back to Oregon, I created a small line of Vegan Bodybuilding & Fitness clothing. I hired a graphic arts student at Oregon State University to come up with the logo for me, and it was great! In fact, I still use the logo on some clothing items today, seven years later. Our primary logo has changed since then. The clothing items became popular from the get-go; we sold t-shirts and a few other clothing items like hats, visors, aprons, and tank tops to people in more than 20 countries and all over North America in just the first couple of years. Since then, we have distributed clothing to people in over 30 countries and from east to west across Canada and the all over the US. I've been able to walk around town and see other people wearing my clothing line. When I attend events like the National Animal Rights Conference, there are sometimes nearly a dozen people on any given day wearing clothing items produced by Vegan Bodybuilding & Fitness. I've seen people on airplanes, at restaurants, at the gym, and around various cities I travel to wearing clothing I produced, and it feels pretty awesome to see this company that I started as a young kid grow because I dedicated my life to making it successful. I still have my clothing produced at the same small business in Corvallis, OR that I initially visited when I got off the cruise ship nearly 8 years ago. Tee's & More Custom Shop has supported me with outstanding service for nearly a decade.

As Vegan Bodybuilding & Fitness grew, our website grew as well. After just a year or two of being primarily focused around me, lots of other vegan athletes started to contact me and tell me about themselves. I immediately incorporated their biographies and featured them on our website with interviews and images. Our online forum grew from a few dedicated members in the early days to nearly 4,000 members today, and it continues to grow. Today, in 2009, we have dozens of vegan athletes featured on our website—dozens of competitive vegan bodybuilders, fitness athletes, and figure models who are getting up on stage like competitive vegan bodybuilder Robbie Hazeley and I—and over 3,500 vegan athletes who are members of our community. There are thousands of others who support us and contribute to the growth of this movement.

After a couple of years of running Vegan Bodybuilding & Fitness, I decided that I was going to film a documentary about vegan athletes. I knew nothing about video production or how I was going to be able to put it all together. But I knew I wanted to do it, and I created a vision and a plan of action to get it done. I contacted various vegan athletes in 2004 and 2005, and by the summer of 2005, I had formed what I called "The Vegan Fitness Team" which consisted of Professional Ironman Triathlete Brendan Brazier, Professional Dancer Tonya Kay, and myself, Amateur Bodybuilder Robert Cheeke. As prominent vegan athletes we set out to make a difference. I produced and directed the documentary in the summer of 2005 with the help from high school friend and college film student Kyle Bucy, and it officially launched in the first months of 2006. Just like our clothing line, it was popular from the day it was announced. Today we have moved thousands of copies to people in more than 30 countries and all over North America. It is on some store shelves for purchase or rent, has been in multiple film festivals, has won awards, and has been the highest grossing project that Vegan Bodybuilding & Fitness has produced to date.

Today Vegan Bodybuilding & Fitness continues to grow. With the up-coming release of the documentary *Vegan Brothers in Iron* and with the release of this book, I see the vegan bodybuilding lifestyle becoming more popular than it has ever been. I go out on tour half the year promoting this lifestyle, growing our online community, and bringing awareness to the movement. It has been a joy of mine to watch this niche industry grow and this grass-roots movement get mainstream exposure. From a website just about me, the only vegan athlete I was aware of, to having more than 3,500 vegan athlete members seven years later is encouraging and very rewarding. These days you can find a Vegan Bodybuilding & Fitness booth at many major vegan festivals throughout the country, and I will likely be at many of them. We sponsor athletes, build communities all over the world, and speak to crowds of vegans and vegetarians and thousands of athletes and people aspiring to improve aspects of their lives as I tour coast to coast throughout the United States every year. We have online muscle contests and opportunities for others to get recognition being featured as one of our profiled athletes on our website. We continue to put out new clothing items, new documentaries and DVDs, and books. The vegan bodybuilding world is growing, and we're here to support the growth of this movement all along the way.

I shared my story of childhood dreams realized, of great bonding experiences with my training partner as we pursued bodybuilding together, and how I built my own company and my own brand based around something I am deeply passionate about. Maybe you're inspired at this point and you want to become a vegan bodybuilder yourself. So where should you to begin? That question is one of the inspirations behind this book, and I am happy to lay some groundwork to help you along in your journey to becoming a vegan bodybuilder.

Before you embark on your new hobby or career as a bodybuilder, here is a list of things to keep in mind to get you started down the road to success:

1. Answer this primary question sincerely: Why are you getting involved in bodybuilding? Then answer the following questions with the same authenticity: What do you plan to achieve as a result of your involvement in bodybuilding? How will bodybuilding benefit you and help you in other areas of your life? Are you ready to make the commitment necessary to live the bodybuilding lifestyle?

2. Once you've established why you want to be involved in bodybuilding in the first place, you'll have a much clearer vision of your upcoming success and everything that it will entail to get there. When you're aware of your desires as a bodybuilder, make a commitment

to the lifestyle. Make it one of consistency and accountability; keep yourself honest every step of the way. If you tell people you train five days a week, make sure you actually train five days a week. If you tell yourself you eat every two or three hours, be sure that you really do eat every two or three hours. Make a commitment and follow through. One of the primary principles that separates successful bodybuilders from unsuccessful bodybuilders is the ability to follow through. Make it happen.

3. Prepare ahead of time. Before you fully embrace bodybuilding as a lifestyle, not just a side project, be prepared for what it will entail. Prepare foods in advance; plan out your day to ensure you will be able to fit in everything you need to do including training, commuting, eating, preparing food, supplementing, and everything else that is involved in the bodybuilding lifestyle. Being prepared will help keep you on course through times of struggle, frustration, and adversity and will help all of your progress come much more smoothly. An easy way to ensure you will always be prepared is to keep a cooler with food in it with you wherever you go and keep non perishable food items like energy bars in your car or backpack so they'll always be with you. If you commute by car, keep a set of workout clothes in your car as well, so no matter where you end up throughout your day, you'll have your gym clothes accessible.

4. Seek advice from people who are experienced and know what they are talking about. Everyone in the gym has their own philosophies, ideas, and opinions about weight lifting, and sometimes their own ideas specifically about bodybuilding too. As in regular life, consider the source of the advice; question where the suggestions are coming from and take all opinions as just that, other people's opinions. Don't fully commit to one set of ideas or principles until you have listened to many different theories so you have the ability to compare ideas and come to a lot of your own conclusions. Trust those who have experienced what you are trying to achieve but ask lots of questions. Anytime you don't know something or don't understand something, ask to get clarification and to have a better understanding, which will help your progress and eventual success. Once you've acquired advice from others, put some of it into action and experiment, taking notes as to which methods yield the best results. There is no single best way to achieve optimal results. Each of us responds differently, so experiment to find what brings out the best in you.

5. Work harder than anyone you know. As in life, the more you put into it, the more you'll get out of it. Work incredibly hard because the rewards, the achievements, and the opportunities that come from intense work ethic will far exceed your expectations. Work hard in the gym; work hard on your nutrition program; work hard on your posing and presentation, and work hard on your commitment to consistency and follow through. Great things will follow. It always works that way. When intention is supported by effort, success follows. Additionally, from a bodybuilding perspective, there is always someone out there working harder than you, and you may be standing next to him or her in your next competition. Turn it up a notch, and make sure you won't get out-worked when you compete. Reveal to everyone in the audience and to your fellow competitors that you have been working extremely hard for a long time for the few moments you have on stage to display it and be rewarded.

6. Visualize what your body will look like and what your life will look like when you achieve your goals. Seeing your future here, in the now, will help keep you working hard day in and day out knowing what successful life lies ahead. This can be one of the most important tools throughout your bodybuilding career. Knowing what you want your future physique and future career to look like and following through everyday to make it a reality is the most empowering action a person can take. As bodybuilders, we get to watch this unfold before our eyes as we transform our bodies to become who we dreamt about.

7. Use tools like vision boards, images of physiques you admire, affirmations, written reminders, motivational quotes and images, and anything else that gets you fired up and motivated to do what you know you have to do in order to be successful. Mapping out your own future in the form of images, phrases, and inspirational words that you are able to see everyday will help reinforce your desires to attain what you set out to achieve. Stay motivated and find what methods work best for you.

8. Seek a support network of people who live a bodybuilding lifestyle and are able to be sympathetic and empathetic of what you are going through. Bodybuilding has its many ups and downs. If you surround yourself with those who have been there or are going through the same things, it makes each situation, each obstacle, that much easier to overcome. Being in communication with other bodybuilders—whether it is at your gym, in your community, or as part of an online community—will naturally increase your support network. It will

help you be part of a community to share advice with and learn from. Use your resources and increase your potential as a result. Always proceed with an open mind and be willing to learn something new.

9. Budget your time and money to have control over the investment that you'll be making to the bodybuilding lifestyle. Understand that there can be many expenses including gym memberships, personal training expenses, increased grocery bills, supplement expenses, tanning sessions, wardrobe changes as your body changes, posing classes, bodybuilding federation membership fees, competition entry fees, cleaning supplies, photography and video fees, preventative and rehabilitative treatment expenses, travel expenses, and lots of other obvious or hidden costs that go along with being a competitive bodybuilder. Understand the monetary commitment that is necessary and budget accordingly. Be aware of the necessary time that will need to be invested as well, which includes commuting to and from your workout facility, training time, additional bathing/shaving time, food preparation time, additional eating time, additional need for sleep or general rest for recovery from training, and other uses of time such as tanning and shopping. There are 1,440 minutes in a day, so you'll need to make adjustments and manage to fit everything in appropriately. Be aware of the increased time you'll need to invest into the bodybuilding lifestyle.

10. Be prepared for changes in your mood as a bodybuilder. Because of the nature of the sport, being one based on image, you'll likely have many psychological ups and downs as you progress, have setbacks, hit plateaus, and have obstacles to overcome. It will affect your overall mood and mindset. Some training sessions will be better than others. Some competitions will be more successful than others. You will go through pre-competition periods of limited diet and increased training. At times you may hit walls; you may want to give up and will have to deal with those situations when you get there. Bodybuilding is an all-day, everyday sport. If it becomes your whole life and you are in a relationship, be prepared to receive a lot of criticism. You will not be spending as much time with your partner as you used to. These are all things to think about because they are all potential realities, but the one thing that is for sure is that your mood will fluctuate as a bodybuilder. It is a natural by-product of living the bodybuilding lifestyle. Keep on going forward, even through the hard times. It will pay off in the end.

As you begin your bodybuilding program always remember what inspired you to become a bodybuilder in the first place, and always remember what bodybuilding means to you. It will help keep your drive alive and your enthusiasm high even when times get tough. When at the end of the day you ask yourself, "Is it worth it?" find a way, every time, to say, "Yes!" If you are able to honestly say that your investment in the bodybuilding lifestyle is worth it because of the fulfillment and reward you get from it, then you are doing better than most people when it comes to contentment in life.

Bodybuilding can be a wonderful part of your life, but it can also be extremely challenging and frustrating. Be prepared for the challenges that lie ahead. It is not all photo shoots, magazine spreads, and attention from peers and trophies. It is a lot of hard work, sometimes injuries and setbacks, and it puts stress on relationships. Bodybuilding by nature is a form of stress on the body and the mind. How you bounce back from those obstacles helps define character and can make you a stronger person at the end of the day—and I'm not just referring to how much weight you can lift. Bodybuilding can easily bring out the best in you and can bring out the worst in you. It all depends on how you handle adversity, stress, and the inherent challenges as well as how you handle the success.

Finding a gym that is convenient and a friend who is interested in bodybuilding too will enhance your overall experience. If you have a romantic partner, suggest that they join you in the gym and make it a joint effort to help bring out the best in each other. Plan out your week of training ahead of time so you won't be tempted to skip workouts and you will be held accountable. Bodybuilding has a unique way of keeping people on track because as soon as you stop training, the results start to go away. That is reason enough to keep on going and to keep improving. Bodybuilding is also a great form of stress relief. Lifting weights and drifting off into your own world of intensity and letting out aggression or frustration on iron is much better than letting out frustration toward people, animals, or objects around the house. Let the gym be a sanctuary for you to be at peace. Let it calm you and ground you and allow you to appreciate everything around you. Let it also be a place for you to unload and explode with intensity through your training.

Begin your bodybuilding lifestyle with an open mind, an open heart, a lot of patience and understanding. With the right discipline and right approach, it could be the sport that teaches you the most about yourself. It's not a team sport. There is nobody else to count on, and you rely heavily on your own will and your ability to gather up the courage to take it on and excel. It's up to you. Is it in you?

Robert's Recap of Beginning Bodybuilding

When you start anything new for the first time, always know why you're doing it and what you hope to accomplish as a result. Weigh out the pros and cons and check in with your heart to see if it is something worth pursuing. Life is extremely short, and you should be doing the things that give you the most fulfillment. Bodybuilding can be one of those things; it has been for me. Most of the greatest days of my life are related to the life that I have created for myself as a vegan bodybuilder. The greatest ways I'm able to contribute are directly related to my outreach as a public figure and vegan bodybuilder, and that means the world to me. But it doesn't mean it's the perfect or ideal lifestyle for you, which is why honestly evaluating your decision to begin bodybuilding is of epic importance.

Bodybuilding isn't easy, and nobody can say that it is, unless they are describing it at its basic level: eat, train, sleep, and repeat. It is easier said than done. Overall, bodybuilding challenges your body and character, making you stronger as a result.

A bodybuilding lifestyle provides countless opportunities because people with a fit and muscular physique are few and far between on a global level. We are a small group and have wonderful opportunities that await us in sports and entertainment. We have the ability to be natural leaders and role models, and we have the power to influence change and make a difference in industries we care about.

Like any other competitive sport or lifestyle, bodybuilding demands commitment and consistency in practice for improvement. Most who aspire to be bodybuilders never make it to the bodybuilding stage because of the challenges that lie ahead and the sheer workload and dedication that it takes. One doesn't have to get on stage to get great fulfillment from bodybuilding and lifting weights, but from experience I can say that competing on stage is one of the greatest levels of fulfillment to be achieved in the sport of bodybuilding.

If a bodybuilding lifestyle is for you and something you want to pursue, then my suggestion is that you go for it with all the enthusiasm you can muster and with a detailed plan in mind. Start slowly, and understand that you have to ease into any new type of athletic training program. Know that results won't happen overnight but will take time and patience. Learn from those who have achieved what you plan to achieve, and ask a lot of questions of those with more experience. Set specific goals and visions for exactly what you want to get out of it and work toward those goals every day and every night until you achieve them. Then, set a higher standard for new visions that will take you to the next level. Enjoy your bodybuilding experience. By nature, bodybuilding has many ups and downs; set out to have far more ups and far more good days. Keep a positive outlook, and those good days will become a reality even through those challenging times. Be safe; have fun; inspire others, and make the most of your opportunity to prove something to yourself and to make a difference through the positive influence you'll have on others.

Robert's Top 10 Reasons to Begin Bodybuilding

1. Bodybuilding will make you a stronger person both mentally and physically.

2. Living a bodybuilding lifestyle gives you something meaningful to work toward everyday.

3. From my experience, because of the work ethic involved in bodybuilding, bodybuilders tend to be more successful in other areas of life that require discipline and focus.

4. Bodybuilding is a way to meet lots of new people from your frequent visits to the gym, when shopping for food, and while interacting with other bodybuilders online and in person at classes and competitions.

5. Bodybuilding is one of the best ways to dramatically improve your physique to something more desirable.

6. The sport of bodybuilding provides lifestyle opportunities you may not have had before. You could be featured on websites and in magazines. You could receive offers to represent companies and products as a result of having a physique that stands out. A variety of unexpected opportunities may arise.

7. A bodybuilding lifestyle gives you one more area of life that is unique that you can refer to and say, "I've done that before." Not many people can say they are bodybuilders; you will be in an elite group.

8. Competing on stage as a bodybuilder is a lot of fun and worth experiencing at least once in your life.

9. Lifting weights regularly will inspire others around you such as your partner, children, parents, or friends to do the same. You'll be helping others get healthier as a by-product of your own efforts in the gym.

10. Weight training can be a very healthy activity to keep your muscles, joints, bones, lungs, and heart in good shape throughout your life.

"There was a point in my life where I felt like I lost all my good friends to drinking and drugs. I felt alone and discouraged. Robert Cheeke's essays and website, www.veganbodybuilding.com, inspired me on so many different levels. It motivated me and made me realize that I should not only be taking care of myself, but improving myself as well. I became motivated to work out, eat healthy, and achieve goals I never thought I would."

Calvin Markus Hagenson
Friend
Phoenix, AZ

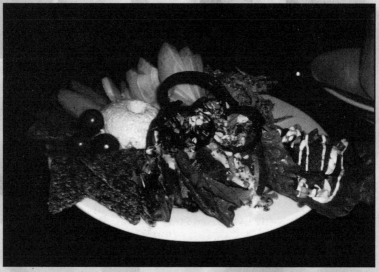

Organic Vegan Cuisine from The Blossoming Lotus, Portland, Oregon

Chapter 3

How to Create a Successful Nutrition Program

Note: I am not a certified dietician, nutritionist or have any formal training in nutrition other than a college course I took many years ago. The information provided is solely based on my experiences and what I have learned as a vegan athlete over the past 14 years. —Robert Cheeke

"Food and nutrition are way more important to gaining mass than training. I mean, you can work out all day, but if you're not feeding the muscle, it's not going to grow."

Victor Martinez
IFBB Pro Bodybuilder,
2007 Arnold Classic Champion

Creating a nutrition program as a bodybuilder is a lot different than creating a nutrition program as a non-bodybuilder. Constructing a nutrition program for a vegan bodybuilder is a whole other story—something quite foreign to most people, including vegans and up-and-coming vegan bodybuilders.

From the onset, one might ask a vegan bodybuilder where he or she gets their protein. Protein consumption is just a singular issue that is given a lot of attention when really there are many components to a sound nutrition program. Protein is at the forefront when it comes to importance and interest among bodybuilders and for good reason: it delivers results, time and time again. But not to be overlooked are the important roles that carbohydrates, fats, and total calories play, not to mention specific vitamins, minerals, and antioxidants as well. Even some non-essential amino acids become "essential" for optimal bodybuilding results based on their functions and contributions to muscle gain, fat loss, and overall health.

Like any quality nutrition program, variety is a major key to overall success. Granted, there are some bodybuilders who eat a very simple, very basic diet for prolonged periods, but I believe that true success in bodybuilding nutrition comes from some variety in diet. It allows for more creativity, enables a bodybuilder to enjoy diversity, and causes less stress emotionally and mentally compared to a very basic diet for which a bodybuilder will lose enthusiasm over time.

Even though variety is an important key to any nutrition program, there are some keys to bodybuilding nutrition that are somewhat unique to the sport and to the lifestyle. Quantity of food becomes a major factor, for example. In a time when many people are looking to cut calories, reduce food intake, cut food costs, and lower their bodyweight, bodybuilders are looking to pour it on. Bodybuilders look to quality and quantity when it comes to their nutrition. I'll be direct right up front. No bodybuilder is going to make any respectable gains on a low protein or low calorie diet. It just doesn't work that way for the majority of athletes, especially bodybuilders. We require a lot of protein and calories to allow ourselves sufficient recovery material and to give our bodies ample opportunity to grow. Unless someone is amazingly genetically gifted and can gain mass and grow muscle without a lot of calories and with only moderate amounts of protein, an aspiring bodybuilder or strength athlete will need to pile on the food in championship style.

I had to learn the hard way because when I started bodybuilding on a vegan diet, I didn't know anyone else in the world doing it. I had to just put ideas into practice and conduct my own trial and error education as a vegan bodybuilder. Like everyone else who lifts weights, I wanted to maximize my gains and give myself the best chance to succeed. Naturally, I turned to standard bodybuilding books and mainstream bodybuilding magazines. I took their advice and "veganized" them. When meals called for high amounts of protein, carbohydrates, and fats, I was there with my vegan food options to answer the call. Luckily there were some things in my favor. I noticed right away that many of the most popular bodybuilding foods among professional bodybuilders were vegan foods, meals that I could eat without having to compromise any morals or ethics to do so. That was highly encouraging, and I was thrilled to realize that some of the absolutely most popular foods among top bodybuilders when polled included, oats, rice, broccoli, yams, potatoes, and vegetables in general. The other foods that topped the list were red meat, fish, eggs, and whey protein, but two of the top three foods were oats and rice. All I had to do was find some "alternatives" to those common high-protein foods frequently recommended to would-be bodybuilders in plant-based form.

For ten years soy was my answer to everything. Soy protein was my answer to whey protein; tofu was my answer to meat, and soy foods in general were my answer to everything from protein powders to protein bars, meals to desserts. It worked well. Aside from the bloating and gas which were annoying by-products, I did gain a lot of strength, put on a lot of muscle, and transformed myself into a bodybuilder. I went from a 120-pound non-vegan teenager to a 190-pound vegan bodybuilder in a relatively short period. I gained 19 pounds over a 12-week period. I kept adding weight and looked like a completely different person from one year to the next as I continued to evolve as a bodybuilder.

Along with the consumption of other popular bodybuilding foods like oats, rice, veggies, and my own favorite foods like fruits, nuts, and pastas, I made a lot of progress. Those who knew me as a skinny teenager were impressed with my gains. After only a couple of years lifting weights I was squatting over 300 pounds, leg pressing over 700 pounds, and pressing 100-pound dumbbells in each hand with ease whether on a flat bench or an inclined bench. I went from a very skinny and thin frame to a much thicker frame closing in on 200 pounds, all built on plant-based vegan foods in just a few years.

I didn't know a lot about nutrition or bodybuilding nutrition back then, but I knew what seemed to work well. I knew I needed to eat…a lot. I knew that eating a lot of calories and protein and being consistent with my training would allow me to reach specific goals that I had for myself. I knew that following the basics that I did understand and doing them well would allow me to overcome some of the things I didn't quite understand about bodybuilding nutrition. I picked what I knew best and did it the best I could. Of course, I had a lot to learn. I was eating as many as 18 tofu hot-dogs in a day trying to get as much protein as possible. My diet wasn't the most exciting it had ever been, but it did work. I ate a lot of pasta, breads, peanut butter, beans, rice, tofu, and up to seven Clif bars a day. I rarely ate green vegetables. I chose to sit rather than stand and didn't like walking or running long distances because I didn't want to burn calories. I was in the game of gaining mass, and I was going to do whatever I could to make it happen, even if it meant years of stomach aches, bloating, and by-passing social activities so I could eat, rest, recover, or train at any hour of the day or night. I worked hard to be the best and wanted it so badly that I did whatever it took, even if it meant stuffing my face full of food until I was sick. I learned a lot from those experiences and not just mistakes that I made. I learned a lot about myself, my will power, my determination, and my passion for excellence.

I ate this way for a long time, from the moment I started bodybuilding to the time I met Professional Ironman Triathlete and fellow vegan Brendan Brazier in 2005. Brendan is the formulator of Vega, the plant-based whole food health optimizer and full line of nutrition products, and he was the person who introduced me to foods I hadn't heard of, though they were common among many plant-based eaters. Brendan had an approach to nutrition that was focused around the consumption of plant-based whole foods. Because of Brendan's influence, I started eating flax seeds, hemp seeds, kale, seaweed, quinoa, some exotic "super foods" like acaí, and a variety of plant-based whole foods I had never tried before. It was a nice change of pace to have some alternatives to soy, which was really my only alternative to meat. After spending time with Brendan and then getting hired by Sequel Naturals, the manufacturers of Vega, I learned more about plant-based whole foods as an approach to eating. I had a lot more variety in my diet as a result. Brendan later wrote *Thrive* and his most recent book *Thrive Fitness*. Brendan has been a great inspiration for me, and his books have been outstanding resources for thousands of people.

We learn by doing, or we learn from other people's influence. In my case, I learned in both ways. I found my own way to success on a vegan bodybuilding diet, and I enhanced it by learning from another vegan athlete who had years of experience and lots of tried, tested, and true knowledge to share. I went from never eating salads to actually wanting to eat salads and even buying salads when going out to dinner when many other options for sandwiches or wraps were available. I stopped drinking natural sodas, something I had been doing for ten years, and started drinking more water, natural and soy-free protein drinks, teas like yerba maté, nutrient-dense smoothies, and real fruit juice. I even started drinking coconut water. I began to buy avocados, seaweed, quinoa, and other healthy foods with names I didn't even know how to pronounce before I met Brendan. Having a friend and a role model who was able to have this kind of influence and impact added so much value to my life and ultimately made me a better athlete, a healthier person, and a better role model for others. I stopped eating soy foods for breakfast, snacks, lunch, dinner, and desserts. I still eat some soy foods. In fact, I like many of them, but I found so many other things to include in my diet that are healthier, more natural, and whole in their unaltered original state, which I think is very important for overall health.

I don't regret the nearly all-soy diet I followed for ten years because it gave me incredible muscle-building gains and it taught me a lot about getting by and making due. Now I eat a wide variety of whole foods, organic foods, fresh foods, soy foods, super foods, and pretty much anything that is vegan.

Though I have cut back dramatically on junk food, I still have some every now and then, and it is enjoyable. But the more my diet improves, the more junk foods become less appealing. Even if there is soy ice cream in front of me or even coconut-based ice cream in the freezer, I'll often pass. I prefer to eat fruits over junk foods any day. I often ask myself, "What will eating this food do for me?" If the answer is a negative or lacking positive benefits, I usually won't eat it.

I give the example of my early vegan bodybuilding diet to show that there are plenty of ways to get to a specific destination, even if your knowledge or resources are limited. If you understand some basics and work hard to apply them everyday, you'll be ahead of most people who are trying to do the same thing. Someone could have an outstanding comprehension of a bodybuilding diet and a background in nutrition but not have the work ethic and desire to put it into practice. That person won't be as successful as the person who understands some basics and puts them into action regularly. Just as you can add muscle eating meat, dairy, and eggs, you can add muscle by eating soy foods or plant-based whole foods as I did. There are many more styles of eating that can also lead to positive results. As long as the proper amounts of calories are consumed with the right ratios of proteins, fats, and carbohydrates and a weight-training program is in place to consistently support it, results will follow. The questions to ask are what is moral, what is ethical, what is in line with your belief system, and what seems to make the most sense and cause the least amount of harm? Eat the foods that are in line with your sincere answers.

Within a compassionate vegan nutrition program, there are still many diet options including processed plant foods, whole foods, raw foods, and a variety of fresh fruits, vegetables, nuts, legumes, grains, and seeds. Those foods consumed with specific quantities and variety will provide your body with the healthy nutrients it needs to thrive and grow. In fact, many will argue that it provides the most powerful form of nutrients because the nutrition is coming from plant-based, whole food original sources. We know the body needs vitamins, minerals, amino acids, fatty acids, and glucose to function, and all of those aspects of nutrition are found in abundance in plant-based whole foods. You wouldn't eat a steak for Vitamin C; you would go to the plant-based whole food sources of Vitamin C to get it. And that can be said for all other vitamins. Fresh plant foods contain everything essential for life and in their best sources. That is just the way nature works. If it comes from nature such as a grain crop, a garden or fruit tree, it is a natural form of food and will contain the highest amounts of nutrients which will support any nutrition lifestyle.

The reason why a lot of people discover that a vegan or vegetarian diet does not work for them is because they don't make "whole foods" the foundation of their nutrition program but rather a lot of processed foods like breads, pastas, processed soy foods, chips, and other junk foods that don't provide much positive nutrition. There is a very clear reason why it doesn't work. I fell victim to this way of eating in my early days as well. When I first became a vegetarian at age 15, my idea of eating a vegetarian diet was having cereal with soymilk, bread rolls, candy, natural soda, chips and salsa, and other junk foods. I nearly gave up on my vegetarian/vegan diet when I was in high school but stuck to it anyway because of my ethics. I learned as I got older to eat healthier foods. I am absolutely convinced that the reason people give up on a vegan diet is because they are not eating healthy foods; namely, they are not eating whole foods. As a result, they may not feel very well, get scared, and go back to eating the poor diet they had before.

Focusing on whole foods gives any diet a better chance for success. A whole food is simply something in its original state. An apple is a whole food; a carrot, a potato, broccoli, cucumbers, tomatoes, berries, etc. are all whole foods. If it grows in the garden, in a field, on a bush, or on a tree, it is a whole food. Foods like bread and potato chips are not whole foods. They are a combination of many food extracts and ingredients, are processed, and not nearly as healthy as something that comes directly from the ground, a bush, or a tree naturally.

Another reason a vegan diet may not work for someone is if they simply don't eat enough food. Many vegans will cut all animal products out of their diet but fail to replace those calories with plant-based foods. Therefore, their caloric intake is reduced, they get thinner, they feel weaker, and decide that a vegan diet isn't for them. In reality, they weren't giving veganism a real chance by eating adequate amounts of proper foods.

If more vegans will incorporate more whole foods into their diets, I guarantee they will feel healthier, feel better, feel more energetic, and feel like a vegan lifestyle is sustainable and worthwhile. Take time to learn on your own. Make a real, honest effort to eat a variety of fruits, vegetables, nuts, grains, legumes, and seeds every day. You will likely be healthier than most people on the planet, assuming you are getting adequate calories throughout the day from sufficient quantity of those whole foods and you are exercising regularly.

Though my diet has changed significantly over my bodybuilding career, I always respect and appreciate each phase I go through and each experience I learn from. Some phases have been healthier than others, more expensive than others, more bizarre than others, more beneficial than others, more cost-effective than others, or more responsible than others; my job is to learn from all my experiences, choose the most beneficial aspects of each phase throughout my nutrition programs, and incorporate them into new programs today. As I extract the benefits from each program, I carry them over to future programs and continue to experience successful results. That is by design, to take what works, discard what didn't work, and try new things along with what has proved to be successful in the past. As 8-time Mr. Olympia winner Ronnie Coleman says, "If you always do what you've always done, you always get what you always got." Sticking to what works and then discovering new things that work well and incorporating them regularly is a recipe for success, and you won't even need to use KC Masterpiece BBQ Sauce like Ronnie uses for this recipe. I suggest doing "more" than what you have "always done" to get superior results. That goes for training and nutrition.

Vegan nutrition and bodybuilding nutrition can be complex on their own, and when you combine the two it becomes even more foreign to most people. When I travel around North America talking about vegan bodybuilding nutrition as I understand it, I talk in very basic terms because I believe it is the basics that are the most important. You don't need to understand the intricate details of a cell or have full comprehension of how carbohydrates get used as fuel or know the conversion rates of specific nutrients. You don't need to name all the steps in ATP Transport or recite the Kreb's Cycle, but if you know what foods to eat, how much to eat, and when to eat them, you will likely find success when you put it into action and follow through with accountability. The further you get into bodybuilding the more scientific you'll probably want to be, but you'll also find out that a lot of it is still the same; it still comes down the basics.

There was a time in my life when I knew quite a bit about nutrition, and I loved it. I loved studying it, understanding it, and having intellectual conversations with people who also understood intricate details of human nutrition. For a time it was a strong interest of mine. Now I rely on the basics of nutrition and rely on conversations with other bodybuilders, or those studying nutrition. Listening, asking questions, talking, and watching those who understand it and put it into action is how I learn about nutrition today. I share from my experiences because I have had success as a vegan athlete, even with my limited knowledge of sports nutrition. I eat every 2-3 hours and focus on consuming healthy foods and find success in my approach. That is all the time and energy I have to devote to it at the moment because of my hectic and excruciatingly busy lifestyle. I also know that pure hard work and application of intense effort will trump knowledge that isn't applied, every time. Would I have more success if I had every aspect of my food consumption carefully evaluated? Perhaps. But not to the degree that I am willing to take on the additional stress in my already stressful life. Some bodybuilders love the scientific approach to weighing and calculating each component of nutritional intake. Some bodybuilders thrive in that environment, carefully measuring just the right amount of rice or oats or protein powder. And to their credit, some have had a lot of success following these methods. I've also used my common sense approach and have placed ahead of these neurotic, compulsive, calculating bodybuilders in competition. It all depends on how far you want to go in the sport, what other passions you have in life, and how you find a way to balance them all out effectively. When it comes to the scientific aspect of bodybuilding nutrition, it is up to the personality of the individual as to which approach they will take. With hard work and dedication, all roads can lead to some form of personal achievement in the sport.

When you become more serious about your bodybuilding program you'll probably become more serious about your nutrition program too. I'm experiencing this at the very moment. I competed more times in 2009 than any other year in my career, and I'm training more consistently than ever. I crave new knowledge to become better, and I seek it out. You'll gain more enthusiasm for the nutrition aspect of bodybuilding just as I am experiencing now. It will become fun and something to really look forward to learning more about. Sometimes this means learning more of the ins and outs of nutrition, including the science behind it to have a better understanding of the role that proteins, fats, and carbohydrates play as well as the role that meal frequency and hydration play in the success of a bodybuilding program. You will be more eager to learn what the best foods are to eat, why they are the best, what they'll do for you, and how you'll benefit from them. You'll want to know more, and more you know the more you'll grow. The better understanding you have of science in general—biology, anatomy, physiology, and nutrition— the more you'll appreciate learning about the scientific aspects of your nutrition program and the more tools you'll have to work with. When you realize how and why the body functions a certain way, you will realize how important food choices are in supporting your body to be at its best. This will give you an incredibly helpful, new perspective on food and will help your bodybuilding lifestyle tremendously. Back when I studied nutrition, kinesiology, anatomy, physiology, and other topics like biochemistry and neurology, it was so much fun because I was just getting interested in bodybuilding at the time. When I understood how carbohydrates were used as fuel and how aerobic and anaerobic fitness impact the body in different ways and what roles different muscles and tendons play and how they work and what makes them signal and function, it became fascinating, and I wanted to learn more. The comprehension of those health aspects isn't necessary for success in bodybuilding, but you may find it worthwhile, helpful, or at the very least interesting to explore the sciences of the human body as you build your own body.

I'm on my 15th year as a vegan athlete and have gone from a skinny kid to an elite endurance runner who placed ahead of two Olympic runners in a race back in 1999, and who ran NCAA collegiate cross country, to a 2-time Northwestern USA Natural Bodybuilding Champion and runner up at the Natural Bodybuilding World Championships in 2006. I've been around the block for a while; I've put in the time, and now I want to do my best to save you some time. I'll share with you what I've learned over the past one and a half decades. Take it for what it's worth; consider the source of the information and see if it fits into your areas of interest.

Here are some Do's and Don'ts I learned over the years about the vegan bodybuilding nutrition program:

DO learn from bodybuilders, nutritionists, dieticians, and those familiar with your lifestyle and bodybuilding goals.

DON'T listen to just any vegan who knows nothing about nutrition or bodybuilders who don't know very much about plant-based nutrition.

DO take the time to learn what the body needs and find out where to get the nutrition it requires from optimal sources.

DON'T just assume you're getting "everything you need" because you follow a vegan diet.

DO eat like a bodybuilder.

DON'T eat like a non-athlete or couch potato.

DO analyze your progress through blood tests, body fat tests, or physicals and make adjustments as time goes on.

DON'T just assume things are working. Get the facts to support your progress.

DO learn as much as you can to support your health and bodybuilding lifestyle.

DON'T conclude that it isn't important to know what to eat and what not to eat.

DO lead by positive example.

DON'T lead by poor example.

DO follow a consistent program to give your body a chance to adapt and improve.

DON'T just eat well during times you feel like it or when it is convenient.

DO ensure there is some sort of variety in your nutrition program that keeps it interesting, rotating staple foods, trying new foods, and experimenting with creativity.

DON'T stay with a stagnant program that lacks excitement and becomes more of a mundane chore than a fun and creative way to support your bodybuilding efforts.

When you make the commitment to creating a sound nutrition program, you're going to first want to know what is required for optimal health and then learn what your options are.

There are many resources out there, and I have searched through some of them to provide you with the following information about required nutrients:

Overview of nutrition, nutrient food sources, and the function of nutrients in the body

Essential nutrients are the carbohydrates, proteins, fats, minerals, vitamins, and water necessary for growth, normal function, and body maintenance. These substances must be supplied by food because most are not synthesized by the body in the quantities required for normal health.[1]

Calories are needed to provide energy so the body functions properly. The number of calories in a food depends on the amount of energy the food provides. The number of calories a person needs depends on age, height, weight, gender, and activity level. People who consume more calories than they burn off in normal daily activity or during exercise are more likely to be overweight.[2]

Protein

Protein is one of the three macronutrients the body uses for energy. One gram of protein provides four calories of energy. Protein is a critical component of a bodybuilding program because it is the component needed to build and maintain large muscle mass. As a general rule, athletes should consume 1-2 grams per pound of bodyweight to build mass and .8-1.5 grams per pound of bodyweight to maintain. Those are standard figures, but everyone is dif-

---

[1] http://medical-dictionary.thefreedictionary.com/essential+nutrients
[2] http://www.nutristrategy.com/nutritioninfo2.htm

ferent so you will want to keep track of your protein consumption to evaluate your own individual protein needs based on your progress and adaptation.

My favorite sources of protein are hemp, pea, rice, beans, lentils, tempeh, tofu, and a variety of grains and greens such as quinoa and spinach. As with all macro and micronutrients, food diversity is key for optimum variety, balance, and overall nutrition. Protein is not a good fuel source and is the least effective form of fuel behind carbohydrates and fats and should be consumed post-workout for its muscle rebuilding and repairing properties. 20 to 50 grams of protein from whole food sources or protein drinks, or a combination of the two is good post-workout protein consumption for the typical bodybuilder. Tailor that quantity range to your own needs. Protein makes up 20% to 40% of my total caloric intake, and I attribute my muscle gains and bodybuilding success to my focus on a high protein bodybuilding nutrition program.

Carbohydrates

Carbohydrates are the main source of energy for the body, providing four calories per gram.

Carbohydrates come in simple forms such as sugars and in complex forms such as starches and fiber. The body breaks down most sugars and starches into glucose, a simple sugar that the body can use to feed its cells.[3] Carbohydrates are found in most foods, and one should be conscientious to choose high-quality carbohydrate sources such as fresh fruits and whole grains for optimal athletic performance. In nearly every athlete's nutrition program, carbohydrates make up the bulk of overall calories, as high as 80% of calories in some athlete's nutrition programs. Eating a wide variety of plant-based whole foods will ensure a diversity of carbohydrates, while also ensuring adequate consumption providing sufficient fuel.

My favorite sources of carbohydrates in general are grains. Brown rice, quinoa, buckwheat, and other grains are excellent sources for sustained energy. I also enjoy popular high-carbohydrate bodybuilding foods such as yams and potatoes. They are staples in nearly every bodybuilder's off season diet to assist with not only fuel, but overall caloric intake and mass.

Immediately before a workout, I carbohydrate-load with a variety of fruit to give me quick, usable energy. Dates, bananas, oranges, apples, grapes, and seasonal berries are my favorite pre-workout foods. Energy bars containing dates and other sugars like agave nectar are also excellent options before a workout. The only time I restrict my carbohydrate intake is in the

---

[3] http://www.medterms.com/script/main/art.asp?articlekey=15381

final weeks leading up to a bodybuilding competition. Aside from those competition preparation periods, I happily welcome large carbohydrate consumption regularly from plant-based whole foods and I suggest that you make them a huge part of your bodybuilding program, perhaps 50% of your calories or more coming from carbohydrates.

Fat

Along with proteins and carbohydrates, fat is one of the three nutrients used as energy by the body. The energy produced by fats is 9 calories per gram.[4]

Fats are needed to keep cell membranes functioning properly, to insulate body organs against shock, to keep body temperature stable, and to maintain healthy skin and hair. The body does not manufacture certain fatty acids (termed essential fatty acids) and the diet must supply these.[5] My favorite sources of essential fatty acids come from flax (omega 3), chia (omega 3) and hemp (omega 3 and 6). I also enjoy eating nuts and a variety of seeds and seed oils for even more variety of quality essential and non-essential fats. Fats are the second best source of fuel behind carbohydrates; therefore, they can be consumed effectively before exercise. Additionally, they have anti-inflammatory properties making them an important part of post-workout nutrition as well.

In general, people tend to consume more omega 6 essential fatty acids than omega 3, so it is important to find quality sources of omega 3 essential fatty acids and incorporate them into your diet regularly. There are non-essential omega fatty acids that have great health benefits too, such as omega 9 fatty acids that can be found easily in pumpkin seeds for example and omega 5 fatty acids found in pomegranates. Though non-essential, they can still provide antioxidants and assist in recovery from exercise, enabling more efficient workouts.

Fats will likely make up 20%-40% of your overall calories.

As you will read later in the chapter, bodybuilders are constantly manipulating the ratio of macronutrient consumption. Balancing the intake of these nutrients is critical for achieving desired bodybuilding results, and a specific program should be customized to each person and each phase of training. If done properly, every aspect of a bodybuilding program from mass-building to pre-contest can be completed with high levels of success. In general, the

---

[4] http://www.medterms.com/script/main/art.asp?articlekey=3394
[5] http://www.answers.com/topic/nutrient

most common macronutrient ratios you're bound to see in a bodybuilding program are likely 50% Carbohydrates, 30% Protein, 20% fats.

In addition to knowing the sources of common and required nutrients, it is also good to know what types of foods to avoid. As I wrote about in *Your Personal Best*, here are some common allergens to know of extracted from that book:

> *It is important to note some of the most common food allergens. I do consume some of them on a regular basis, and each person's response to them is totally individually based. Some people can tolerate all common allergens; some can't tolerate any.*

> *The most common allergen foods according to www.foodallergy.org (which are the same commonly accepted allergens throughout North America) are:*

Common Food Allergens

> *Cow's milk (Dairy products)*
> *Eggs*
> *Peanuts*
> *Tree Nuts*
> *Fish*
> *Shellfish*
> *Soy*
> *Wheat*

> *Four of the eight most common allergens I avoid naturally, as they are animal derived, and the others are ones that even if I consume regularly, I pay attention to my body's reaction, if any, and then make my future decisions regarding those foods accordingly.[6]*

Creating a nutrition program is an essential part of a successful bodybuilding program. Deciding what type of bodybuilding program you want to follow is up to you. There are various approaches based on goals and what is being attempted. There are various "seasons" throughout bodybuilding that all require different diets. Some people have wildly different diets from season to season, and others eat the same way year-round with slight modifications to fit the specific time of year or theme of preparation.

---

[6] Robert Cheeke, *Your Personal Best,* 224.

Here are some fairly common themes in bodybuilding nutrition:

- Mass-Building Nutrition Program (sometimes called off-season diet)
- Fat-Burning Nutrition Program (sometimes called cutting-up diet or leaning-out diet)
- Pre-Contest Nutrition Program (usually called pre-contest diet)
- Maintenance Nutrition Program (considered an everyday maintenance diet)

It has to be clarified that there is a difference between eating for health and eating for athletic performance, for muscle growth, or for mass gain, especially in bodybuilding. Many think they go hand-in-hand—eating for athletic performance must also mean eating for health. But that isn't how it always works in the world of bodybuilding. A bodybuilding diet is much higher in protein, carbohydrates, fats, fluids, and supplements than that of the average healthy person. One could argue that aspects of a bodybuilder's nutrition program are in fact unhealthy, and it is a valid argument. The point of bodybuilding isn't to be as healthy as possible, but it is to build a physique that is in the best possible shape based on what judges are looking for in the *sport* of bodybuilding, or based on what you are looking to get out of life based on your physique. It is to look your very best in relation to muscle size, symmetry, balance, and conditioning and doesn't focus on "health" as its primary objective.

An animal-based bodybuilding diet—one of consuming meat, eggs, dairy, and other animal products—has historically been extremely unhealthy for bodybuilders based on the sheer quantity of meat and other high cholesterol and saturated fat-laden foods that are consumed. Many bodybuilders suffer from clogged arteries, off-season and post-career obesity, and have a myriad of other health-related problems often having to do with heart trouble. This is a known risk all bodybuilders take, and so many of them suffer the effects of their long-time heavy animal-based diet to achieve something in their sport that they think is only attainable on an animal-based diet.

Vegan bodybuilders are better off simply because they are not taking in the high cholesterol foods. They also usually consume less saturated fats, toxins, and acid-forming foods and focus more on plant-based whole foods— food from the earth, fields, bushes, and trees. Though not as unhealthy as an animal-based bodybuilding diet, a vegan bodybuilding diet can be unhealthy as well based on the high amounts of calories, protein, and processed foods often consumed. The manipulation of specific components of nutrition, for example the yo-yoing of high and low carbohydrates and water intake, is tough on the body, but it helps the bodybuilder fulfill his or her bodybuilding goals. Luckily, many of these intentional unhealthy behaviors are short lasting and temporary and usually don't have dramatic or severe adverse implications on overall or long-term health. However, repetition over time can have long lasting negative health implications and is something that should be considered by everyone who is involved in bodybuilding and who follows a bodybuilding diet.

One of the visions behind this book is to show non-vegan athletes and bodybuilders that there is a healthier way to live their lifestyle, therefore prolonging their life and creating a higher net gain quality of life without having to jeopardize their bodybuilding or athletic dreams or success.

Bodybuilders, vegan or not, are faced with a double-edged sword when it comes to health and their bodybuilding careers. We have to follow some perceived unhealthy habits in order to achieve our goals and dreams within the world of bodybuilding. Even our intense, hardcore workouts could be described as unhealthy based on the impact they have on our joints, muscles, tendons, and the toll it takes on our bodies. We do the same nutritionally as we stuff our faces full of food, pump our bodies full of protein powders and supplements, and then starve ourselves, deplete ourselves of water, and take other drastic measures as we prepare to get on the bodybuilding stage. At times we're playing with fire, and we know it. But we do it to chase dreams and to live outstanding lives with high levels of personal fulfillment and satisfaction.

Many of us do monitor our progress, are aware of our risks, and take precautions to make our bodybuilding lifestyle as healthy as we can. When I know I've gone too long without water or when I've been on a low carbohydrate diet too long, I make changes so I can feel better and take care of my body. For the most part, it's all short-term adaptations we make to achieve a certain look for a brief period of time. We don't put ourselves at health risks year-round, but rather weeks at a time before competition. We all handle the nutrition aspect of bodybuilding differently. Some pay very close attention to it and make every effort possible to be as healthy as possible. Others don't worry very much about health and focus on getting every bodybuilding benefit possible. Some will claim they "listen to their body," but sometimes symptoms and problems don't show up until later in life, so I would never fully rely on "listening to your body." We're usually battling dehydration or muscle cramps, both which can be remedied pretty quickly. If you ever question whether you have any health-related issues as a result of bodybuilding, I suggest getting checked out right away. Your body can tell you some things, but not everything, so periodic health check-ups are something I'd recommend.

I was recently asked by a couple of doctors why I pursue a high protein diet when I know it stresses the kidneys. The doctors were perplexed and confused and asked, "Why would you want to get bigger?" Suggesting it was an issue of vanity. I explained to them that I do what I do so I can reduce animal suffering by leading as a positive role model through a vegan bodybuilding lifestyle to show that it is possible, practical, and attainable on a pure plant-based diet. I also really enjoy my bodybuilding lifestyle. I don't fear that my protein intake is so high that it is causing problems. I have had blood work done to monitor the levels, and I'll get blood work done again to ensure I am okay. If at anytime I experience measurable adverse health problems from my bodybuilding nutrition program, I'll make some changes, but until then I will move full speed ahead, adding mass to my frame and making a massive difference in the world.

As bodybuilders, many of us are concerned about potential health risks. We do pay attention to them, take them seriously, and take precautions when needed. Some precautions include an increase in water consumption. We do this to support our kidneys which work overtime to process all the protein we eat on a regular basis. Kidneys process protein just as the liver processes alcohol for example. A high protein diet does tax the kidneys and other organs involved in the transportation, delivery, storage, and usage of protein in the body. Taking in additional fluids, especially water, can help reduce the stress put on the organs to some degree. It makes sense to stay well hydrated all the time, except in the final days before competition when we deliberately dramatically reduce hydration in order to reveal more definition in our bodies.

As vegan bodybuilders, we're still likely healthier than 95% of the global population and not just because over 50% of the global population is malnourished or obese, but because we are fairly healthy most of the time and focus heavily on plant-based whole foods. I personally don't believe that my total calorie and protein consumption is having dramatic adverse effects on my health. Overall, I see my diet as basically fueling my body for my athletic performance allowing me to recover, grow, and improve while enabling me to live my desired lifestyle saving lives and inspiring many. My bodybuilding nutrition program, including my mass-building nutrition programs, fuel my success and allow me to achieve dreams which gives me so much personal fulfillment, it seems worth it every time.

Mass-Building Vegan Bodybuilding Nutrition and Meal Programs

A mass-building vegan bodybuilding program can be a lot of fun. Of all the areas of bodybuilding nutrition, mass-building is probably my favorite. I can eat pretty much whatever I want, in whatever quantities I want. I gain weight and can lift much heavier weights in the gym simply because I have more overall mass to move the weight with. The increase in my bodyweight along with my total calorie and protein consumption allow me to get bigger and stronger. This nutrition program is something I look forward to every year. It is a time when I am at my best even when I don't "look" like I'm at my best since I'm carrying more body fat, have less definition, and don't bother with fake tans. But I really do feel at my best because I'm at my strongest, and I'm watching progress take place before my eyes. I've created pages on my website titled, "Losing definition and loving it." I enjoy being ripped and covered in veins too, but there is nothing like a thick, solid, dense, muscle-bound physique, and someday I plan to own one year round.

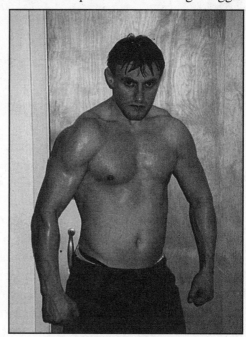

Robert age 23 at 193 pounds
(photo by Eric Brown)

Some general tips for bulking up on a mass-building vegan bodybuilding diet

<u>Eat Plenty of Protein</u>

You will need to eat lots of protein. That is all there is to it. Forget what the agencies and administrations say about recommended daily intake; that is for average people and certainly doesn't apply to bodybuilders. You will likely need to consume 1-2 grams of protein per pound of bodyweight if you have any aspirations of adding muscle or even maintaining the muscle you've worked hard to build. If you are a 200-pound bodybuilder, consuming 35-50 grams of protein at a time, six times a day should easily keep you on course for muscle growth. Combine that with adequate consumption of carbohy-

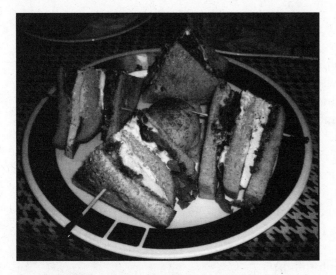

Southeast Vegan Club Sandwich from Hungry Tiger Too in Portland, Oregon

drates and fats, and you should be well on your way to adding mass, bulking up, and achieving your bodybuilding goals. Once you figure out the best foods to eat to reach those targets, it won't seem difficult or challenging but will become second nature. If your work ethic and your training programs support your sound nutrition programs, your results will be even greater.

There is a lot of talk about low-protein diets in the general health community and especially in the vegan community. This focus on low protein consumption is sound advice for the typical inactive person and non-athlete. Those people simply don't require large quantities of protein to be healthy, and I fully support this notion of a low to moderate protein diet for the average inactive or low activity person. But when we're talking bodybuilding and strength and power sports, a high protein diet is required for success. It is very hard to build muscle on low protein diets, even when the protein sources are of high quality. I have experimented with low-protein diets, and thousands of bodybuilders experiment with various quantities of protein intake every day. Nearly all of us come to the same conclusion—the body responds best to high protein and adequate calories when repairing and building muscle.

Every time my protein intake has been at its highest, I have experienced the best muscle-building results. There is no question about that. I've documented for years that a high-protein and high-calorie diet brings out the best in my physique. I have over 100 pages of documented nutrition journal entries to back up my results. Conversely, every time I have lowered my protein intake to a standard amount, I experience inferior mass-building results. In some cases I wasn't even able to hang on to the muscle mass I already had.

Once I increase my protein consumption to 1-2 grams per pound of bodyweight a day, I build muscle and add size again. I also feel like I am at my psychological best when I am taking in large amounts of protein. I honestly feel that I am treating my muscles well and giving them a real chance to grow and adapt and recover from weight training sessions when I am feeding them high amounts of protein. It not only makes me feel really good mentally, physically, and psychologically, but also prevents me from feeling bad, inadequate, or paranoid. I have experimented over the years and found that those early days of very high protein and high total calories were the most effective methods I've ever used for adding muscle through nutrition. In fact, even with my new knowledge of all kinds of great foods to incorporate into my diet, I often refer back to the early days and turn to the foods that pumped me up quickly, which were very high in protein. For me, it really does make a significant difference, and I love giving myself the best opportunity to succeed no matter what I'm doing.

In this chapter I have included five mass-building nutrition programs as well as some of my "real" mass-building programs taken directly from my nutrition diary from my early years as a growing bodybuilder. It is fun to look back years later and see where my dedication was apparent, what my diet was like, and observe and re-read the steps I took in order to make serious progress. I will also list my all-time favorite mass-building foods which may serve as a good resource for you to extract some ideas to incorporate into your own nutrition program. The truth is, for years I was embarrassed to reveal what I "really ate" when I went through the most successful bulking phase of my bodybuilding career. Some of the foods honestly aren't the healthiest foods in the world, but the total dedication to high protein and high calories in my diet made all the difference and made my results possible. So even though I'm not always proud of some of the foods I ate (such as up to 18 tofu hot dogs in a day or 12 bagels in a day for example). I am proud of the gains that I made and proud of the success that followed and the incredible bodybuilding lifestyle that ensued. I'm putting all the cards on the table revealing my past diet, my current diet, and the highlights of the past ten years while on a mission to bulk up from the skinny farm boy to pro-wrestler, real-life version of He-Man.

April 16, 2003

Meal #	Time	Food	Protein	Calories	Water	Notes
1	7:30 AM	Cereal w/ soymilk / Orange juice	11 / 2	300 / 110		
2	10:00 AM	oatmeal bar	7	250	17oz	
3	11:15 AM	oatmeal bar	7	250	17oz	
4	12:30 PM	4 tofu hotdogs / bread / mango / strawberries / orange juice	52 / 7 / 1 / 2	240 / 200 / 150 / 110		
5	2:30 PM	orange / bread	1 / 3	80 / 150		
6	4:00 PM	oatmeal bar	7	250	17oz	
7	5:00 PM	banana / 2 tofu hotdogs / strawberries	2 / 6 / 1	90 / 160 / 150	17oz	
8	6:00 PM	2 soy protein drinks / multivitamin wellman pill(s)	28 / —	260	17oz	
9	6:30 PM	tofu hotdog / bread / strawberries	13 / 7 / 1	80 / 200 / 150	17oz	
10	7:30 PM	2 hot hotdogs / bread / papaya enzymes	26 / 7	160 / 200	17oz	
11	9:30 PM	walnuts	7	170	17oz	
12	10:00 PM	Baked tofu	40	300	17oz	
13	11:00 PM	Soy protein drink / strawberries	14 / 1	120 / 80	60oz	
			268	4,260	163	

It's My time now
to get HUGE

18-20-00	grot protein	calories
Clif bar	12	240
Bagel	11	320
Juice	4	240
Tofu hotdog	9	45
Bread	4	90
tofu hotdog + bread	13	135
tofu hotdog	9	45
Spaghetti Sandwich	9	200
Bagel w/peanut butter	18	500
tofu turkey sandwich	8	225
fruit smoothie	2	100
Peanuts	8	200
Strawberry protein drink	10	300
Soy delicious	2	130
Bagel & peanut butter	18	500
tofu hotdog	9	45
fruit smoothie	2	100
peanuts	12	300
Chocolate soy milk	10	250
tofu hotdog & bread	13	135
	183	4,100

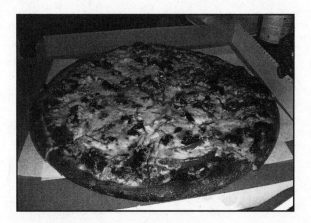

*Vegan Pizza from
Peace O Pie in
Boston, MA*

<u>Be prepared to defend yourself</u>

When you're on a high-protein diet, be prepared to defend your high-protein consumption choices, especially among other vegans or those in the general health community. You will need to express the bodybuilding and personal fulfillment benefits you get from your high protein diet clearly so it is easily understood. You may have to admit that it is not exclusively a health decision but also one that is not profoundly unhealthy. You may be inclined to explain that it is an athletic performance decision that supports your personal and career interests. It is quite likely that the people who criticize your high-protein diet don't have similar goals and may not fully understand your desire and your commitment. Most people don't know what it is like to work hard to achieve something outstanding in the athletic realm, especially in the sport of bodybuilding. The odds aren't in your favor for having people understand your mass-building desires as we live in a society of obesity where most people desire to lose size not gain. You may not run into many confrontations at all, but it is something to be conscious of, especially in the vegan community where eating high amounts of protein and calories and pushing heavy weights around usually isn't on the daily schedule. Do what is most comfortable, what gives you the best results, and what makes the most sense to you. Stand up for yourself and defend your decisions. I stand by my decisions whether people agree with them or not, and it is empowering. I'm not always the most popular person in the room when I voice my opinion, but I'm often one of the most athletically accomplished in the room and have the most fulfillment from my athletic lifestyle and that is good enough for me. When you do take a stand and defend your position and explain why you do what you do, you could very easily inspire a lot of people and change their ways of thinking. Leaders always do that. When you lead by example with confidence, you are bound to have followers who admire your work ethic, desire, and accomplishments and who respect the direction you are heading.

Having records of prior success will help when defending your nutrition choices. Record your meal programs so you have something to reflect back on, just as I am doing now as I review my old mass-building programs from ten years ago. Be confident in your decisions and observe how your body responds. If it responds well, keep doing what works and record it. Having a physique superior to others in the bodybuilding sense speaks volumes. There is no better defense than displaying those achievements on your physique for people to see first-hand. When your physique stands out enough, you won't have to defend your decisions because your body will do the talking for you.

Keep your total caloric intake high

Just as important as ingesting large amounts of protein is the consumption of a high total calorie diet. To be a successful bodybuilder this is a necessary evil. Bodybuilding is a physically demanding sport. The muscles, joints, and tendons need calories to recover from the intense training. Eating a high protein diet will help considerably with this effort because many high protein foods are also high calorie foods such as almond butter, nuts and seeds, grains, protein powders, etc. However, the majority of calories will come from carbohydrates because nearly every plant-based food is packed full of them, and they are necessary to provide expendable energy. Even though they are lower in calories, whole foods like fruits and vegetables should be consumed daily for the health benefits, especially their vitamin, mineral, and anti-oxidant contents.

A 200-pound bodybuilder will likely want to consume 4,000-6,000 calories a day to add mass. It may seem like a lot of food, and it is, but for an athlete of that size, that amount of calorie consumption is necessary to improve athletic performance. Heavy weight training creates micro-tears in muscles, and the body needs calories, especially specific amino acids such as L-glutamine, Branched-chain Amino Acids (BCAA's), and protein in general, to rebuild and replenish and prevent injury.

Don't be afraid to eat big. If you want to get big you have to eat big. If you want to be a champion, you have to eat like a champion. If you work out enough, you will be hungry and eating won't seem like a chore. Eating has been a chore for me when I'm sitting around trying to pack in calories, but when I'm training for an hour or two a day with high intensity and when I'm doing aerobic exercise like running or playing basketball or soccer, I get really hungry and I can eat a lot more. Eat smaller meals throughout the day and you'll see that over the course of the day, the calories really add up. Your largest meals will likely be breakfast, lunch, dinner, and post workout. With six to eight meals a day, half being larger and half being smaller, you can balance out a solid nutrition program to fuel your body with what it needs to thrive. It may take time for the body to adapt to an increase in calories so a typical approach is to ease into it, adding a few hundred calories per day each week. If you are currently consuming 2,500 calories a day, next week bump it up to 2,800 calories a day, and every week thereafter take it up another 300 calories until you reach a sufficient level for optimal muscle growth, which will likely be somewhere between 4,000 and 7,000 calories depending on your gender, size, activity level, etc. This will allow your body to adapt to the increased workload of consuming, processing, using, and eliminating the extra calories. It is more of a shock on the body to try to go from 2,500 to 5,000 calories a day overnight, and in fact, I wouldn't recommend it. Ease into it just as a runner eases into endurance training. Take your time; choose your favorite foods, and allow your body to adapt to the changes. Take small, deliberate steps to allow your body to adapt naturally, just as it adapts to increased workloads in the gym.

One tip that helps a lot of people gain mass is to consume liquids such as protein drinks for quick consumption of calories, fast absorption and assimilation of nutrients, and lower stress on the digestive system. This really is one of the best ways to approach an increase in calories. It's so much easier to eat an entire bag of spinach if it is blended, for example, than to eat it leaf by leaf out of a bag or from the garden. The same goes for any food. You can blend up five whole pears and consume them more easily than consuming five whole pears bite by bite. As I was leading up to recent bodybuilding competitions, I was drinking as many as eight low-carbohydrate protein drinks a day. By doing so, I had great bodybuilding results from the liquid calories. I placed in the top three in three out of four competitions during that spring competition run, including one first place finish. Some of my photos ended up in major print media—Alicia Silverstone's book The Kind Diet, for example. Some of the images taken of me in my bodybuilding form during that period are my most frequently used images in my current media outreach.

Review my mass-building nutrition programs and lists of mass-building foods listed at the end of this section to help support your progress. Combine your nutrition efforts with mass-building compound exercises, and you'll be sure to turn some heads and take steps toward achieving your bodybuilding physique and lifestyle goals.

Consistency of training and nutrition

I honestly believe that consistency is the most important key to success. I've even said that it is the most important word, period. One cannot achieve anything without consistency of applied effort. The more consistent someone is, the more success they are bound to have. If you hope to put on muscle, you will have to put in the work consistently with your training and nutrition programs or you simply won't achieve what you set out to do. Success simply isn't possible if you don't adhere to consistency to see it through. It is a physiological impossibility to put on muscle without consistency in good nutrition and training programs. That is just the way the body works. Sure, some of us adapt faster than others based on our genetic make-up, and patience will likely play a role in your eventual success. But largely it is the people who put in the time day in and day out, grinding through their workouts and sticking to their eating program, who stand out and adapt, improve and succeed, all as a result of their dedication to consistency.

This dedication to consistency is mandatory for achieving results you are looking for as a bodybuilder and is a prerequisite for success in life. If you enjoy weight training and enjoy eating, then it won't feel like a burden for you to do those things everyday in sufficient quantities. Rather, it will be fun, motivating, rewarding, and something you look forward to daily. Sometimes there are aspects of your vision that you want to attain that will be a chore and a burden, but when you understand the big picture and realize that they are part of the process that leads to the eventual achievement that will provide high levels of personal fulfillment, you will do them anyway. Not every single aspect of achieving a goal is fun, enjoyable, and inspiring. Sometimes, it's downright challenging. That is when you challenge yourself and demand more from yourself and find out what you're really made of—if you have what it takes to rise to the occasion. If you can gather up the courage to say, "Yes I can" even when times get tough and when aspects of the process of attainment become a burden, you better yourself and prove to yourself that you can overcome and achieve, and it helps you become stronger in other areas of life.

Now that you have read through the different aspects of mass-building and know why and how you're going to approach this quest, I have provided the following meal programs to be used as guidelines to get ideas for your own mass-building nutrition programs. You don't need to follow these exactly to get desired results. In fact, I wouldn't even suggest you follow them exactly. Many are very bland and redundant because that is how I eat. I eat for functionality, not to please my palate, though many of the foods I suggest are quite popular among most audiences and I think you'll get something worthwhile out of reading them. These programs are simply samples that I have come up with based on my own experiences over the years. As stated at the beginning of the chapter, they have not been approved by the FDA or any other health governing body, and you should consult a physician or nutrition-ist before following any of the guidelines put forth.

Most of my meal programs throughout this book are based on six meals a day, but for mass building I have made these to reflect eight meals a day. When I am mass building, I really do eat eight times a day, if not more.

Mass-building Meal Programs

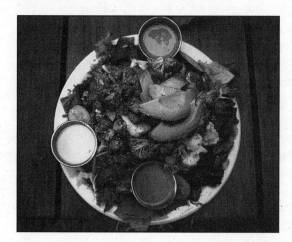

Large protein salad with tofu, avocado, seeds and a variety of greens from Nearly Normals Vegetarian Restaurant – Corvallis, OR

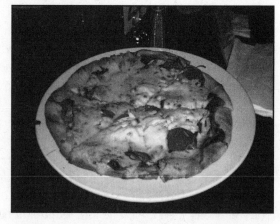

Vegan pizza from Ethos Vegan Kitchen – Orlando, FL

Mass-Building Meal Program #1

Meal #1
>3 large vegan pancakes with maple syrup or vegan butter (or both)
>12 ounces of orange juice
>Protein drink

Meal #2
>2 protein bars
>2 whole fruits
>Protein drink
>16 ounces of water

Meal #3
>2 large burritos
>12 ounces of fruit juice
>16 ounces of water

Meal #4
>2 whole fruits
>Vega meal replacement drink
>16 ounces of water

Meal #5
>2 tofu sandwiches with avocado
>16 ounces of fruit juice
>16 ounces of water

Meal #6
>Bowl of quinoa, broccoli, carrots, peas, peppers, and tofu
>Large green salad with nuts and seeds and Vega omega 3-6-9 EFA oil
>Protein drink
>16 ounces of water

Meal #7
>2 almond butter sandwiches
>16 ounces of hemp milk
>16 ounces of water

Meal #8
>   A collection of vitamin supplements (Vitamin B-12, Omega 3
>   and 6, multivitamin, etc.)
>   2 whole fruits
>   Green smoothie with fruits and protein

Estimated Totals:
>   Total Calories = 6,850
>   Total grams protein = 300g
>   Total grams of carbohydrates =1200g
>   Total grams of fats = 80g
>   Total water consumption = 150 ounces (factoring in water for
>   protein drinks too)

Mass-Building Meal Program #2

Meal #1
>   Plate of tofu scramble with potatoes, peppers, broccoli, and other
>   veggies
>   2 veggie sausages
>   2 slices of bread with almond butter or jam
>   12 ounces of orange juice
>   16 ounces of water

Meal #2
>   2 pieces of whole fruit
>   2 cups non-dairy yogurt
>   Protein drink
>   16 ounces of water

Meal #3
>   Bowl of whole wheat pasta with pinto beans
>   Large green salad
>   16 ounces of water

Meal #4
>   Plate of vegetables with hummus dip
>   4 slices of pita bread with lentil paté
>   16 ounces of water

Meal #5

Bowl of brown rice with broccoli and asparagus
Avocado and sprouts sandwich
Large green salad
16 ounces of water

Meal #6

Protein drink
3 yams
Large bowl of vegetable soup
16 ounces of water

Meal #7

Rice and vegetable stir-fry with baked tofu
Small bowl of kale leaves
16 ounces of hemp milk
16 ounces of coconut water

Meal #8

2 pieces of whole fruit
Green protein smoothie with Vega Smoothie Infusion
A bowl of coconut ice cream

Estimated Totals:

Total Calories = 7,000
Total grams protein = 350g
Total grams of carbohydrates =1100g
Total grams of fats = 130g
Total water consumption = 150 ounces (factoring in water for
protein drinks too)

Mass-Building Meal Program #3

Meal #1

Breakfast burrito
Bowl of fried potatoes
16 ounces of grapefruit juice
16 ounces of water

Meal #2

> 2 high protein food bars (Vega Bar, PROBAR, Clif Bar, Organic Food Bar, others)
> 3 non-dairy yogurts
> Fruit smoothie with protein and greens
> 16 ounces of water

Meal #3

> Large plate of Pad Thai with noodles, veggies, tofu, and peanut sauce
> 2 cups of brown rice
> Small green salad
> 16 ounces of water

Meal #4

> Protein drink
> 3 pieces of whole fruit
> 2 servings of walnuts
> 16 ounces of water

Meal #5

> Five slices of vegan pizza
> Small green salad with Vega omega 3-6-9 EFA oil
> 16 ounces of hemp milk
> 16 ounces of water

Meal #6

> Green protein smoothie
> 2 almond butter and jam sandwiches
> 16 ounces of water

Meal #7

> Large spinach pie
> Middle Eastern food platter with garbanzo beans, lentils, hummus, rice, etc.
> 4 slices of pita bread for dipping in the platter
> 16 ounces of water

Meal #8

> 2 slices of vegan chocolate cake with vegan ice cream
> Small bowl of assorted fruit
> Protein drink

Estimated Totals:
>Total Calories = 8000
>Total grams protein = 315g
>Total grams of carbohydrates = 1200g
>Total grams of fats = 200g
>Total water consumption = 130 ounces (factoring in water for protein drinks too)

Mass-Building Meal Program #4

Meal #1
>Large bowl of oats with Vega meal replacement powder
>   Protein smoothie
>Whole wheat bagel with vegan cream cheese
>16 ounces of water

Meal #2
>2 tofu sandwiches on sprouted bread
>Medium green salad with Vega omega 3-6-9 EFA oil
>Protein drink
>16 ounces of water

Meal #3
>Veggie taco platter with beans, tomato, avocado, lettuce, rice, and tortillas
>Green protein smoothie
>16 ounces of water

Meal#4
>Green salad with Field Roast Grain meat
>Bowl of dates rolled in coconut flakes
>Protein drink
>16 ounces of water

Meal #5
>Tempeh Reuben sandwich
>Bowl of chips and salsa
>Small bowl of lentil soup
>16 ounces of water

Meal #6
> Large bowl of sliced assorted fruits
> Green protein smoothie
> 16 ounces of water

Meal #7
> 2 baked potatoes with seitan, broccoli, carrots, and almond gravy
> Green salad with hemp seeds, seaweed, and Vega omega
>   3-6-9 EFA oil
> 16 ounces of water

Meal #8
> Bowl of chocolate tofu pudding with strawberries
> 12 ounces of rice milk
> 2 pieces of fruit
> 8 ounces of water

Estimated Totals:
> Total Calories = 7,500
> Total grams protein = 300g
> Total grams of carbohydrates =1100g
> Total grams of fats = 200g
> Total water consumption = 170 ounces (factoring in water for
> protein drinks too)

Mass-Building Meal Program #5

Meal #1
> 3 pieces of French toast with maple syrup
> Bowl of cereal with rice milk
> 2 pieces of whole fruit
> 16 ounces of water

Meal #2
> Vega meal replacement drink
> 2 pieces of whole fruit
> 1 Protein bar
> 16 ounces of water

Meal #3

6 vegan corndogs
Medium green salad with Vega omega 3-6-9 EFA oil
16 ounces of water

Meal #4

1 large cucumber with hummus
3 large carrots
Green Protein Smoothie (Vega Smoothie Infusion)
16 ounces of water

Meal #5

Plate of steamed vegetables with tempeh
Green salad with seaweed and hemp seeds
An assortment of nuts
16 ounces of water

Meal #6

Celery sticks with almond butter
2 pieces of whole fruit
Protein bar
16 ounces of water

Meal #7

Kale salad with dulse and pumpkin and hemp seeds
Green Smoothie with Vega Smoothie Infusion
16 ounces of water

Meal #8

2 oranges
Plate of flax crackers with almond butter
12 ounces of water

Estimated Totals:

Total Calories = 7,750
Total grams protein = 300g
Total grams of carbohydrates =1275g
Total grams of fats = 160g
Total water consumption = 170 ounces (factoring in water for
protein drinks too)

I admit the calorie totals seem a little outrageous, but nearly everything about mass-building bodybuilding is outrageous, including the physiques of those who do it right. The totals are just estimates based on the foods listed, and the foods listed are just suggestions that model some of the meals I ate when I was consuming over 5,000 calories a day. They may look intimidating, but take whatever you want from the meal programs and see how it fits into your current mass-building program. If you're not seeing the results you're looking for, you're probably not eating enough or training enough, or you simply don't care enough. What will you do to change what you're doing now in order to get where you're trying to go? How badly do you want to grow and improve?

Robert's all-time favorite mass-building foods are the following:

> Tofu
> Tempeh
> Seitan
> Nuts
> Nut butters (peanut butter, almond butter, etc.)
> Avocado
> Beans
> Brown rice
> Quinoa
> Pastas
> Sandwiches
> Burritos
> Soups
> Artisan breads
> Protein bars
> Protein drinks
> Heavy foods by weight such as potatoes and yams
> Ethic food platters such as Middle Eastern, Thai, Indian and
>   Ethiopian foods

Fat Burning – Toning up and leaning out

One of the most common statements people make when talking to me about fitness is that they want to "tone up" their body or "lean out" or "get cut up." These expressions are all professing the same desire. It basically means they want to have lower body fat and better muscle definition. Some have a desire to reveal abdominal muscles hiding behind a layer (or many layers) of fat, or see lines in their arms from muscle separation of biceps, triceps, and shoulders, or improve the muscle tone in their legs and glutes; others want to alter their overall shape, drop body fat in general, and be in better physical condition. Any way you describe toning up, the idea is to burn fat to achieve the desired outcome of looking fit.

   The first requirement of burning fat and toning up is to reduce processed, refined, and sugary foods from the diet that caused fat storage in the first place. Why not eliminate the source right from the beginning to have less work to do later on? Refined foods are the types of foods that make the body store the most fat, so it makes practical sense to reduce or eliminate them all together. One of the

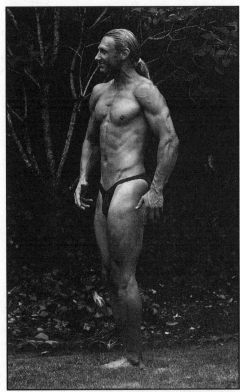

Photo by Randall Perez – RandallPerez.com

best ways to reduce those fat-building foods is to replace them with fresh whole foods like fruits and vegetables. Fruits and vegetables are lower in calories, more natural, contain more water, and most importantly, don't contain the bad sugars and processed ingredients that refined foods and junk foods contain. Taking fat-burning pills and supplements help to some degree but certainly are not the most natural way to go and may have some dangerous side effects. Rather than relying on pills, rely on accountability; clean up your diet to reflect the desire to improve your physique, drop body fat, and increase visible muscle tone. Improvements in nutrition and training programs are always going to be the best ways to achieve fat burning within the body. It's up to you to implement the positive changes whenever you're ready to start seeing results. As always, I suggest now as the best time to start.

   A lot of diet programs have "cheat days" where you can eat whatever you want from pizza to burgers. But that has never made a whole lot of sense to me. If those foods are known for contributing to fat storage and your goal is to reduce body fat, it isn't a sensible plan to follow, even if it is only once per week or very seldom. This concept of "cheat days" to eat junk food is still counter-productive to your entire objective and should be avoided. "Cheat days" also invite some negative patterns to develop such as "cheat days" in other areas of life from skipping out on school to missing meetings which is one more reason why they should be avoided. If your goal is to build mass, it's totally acceptable to have a cheat day, but if your goal is to burn fat, show some accountability to support your ambitions. Quit cheating your way out of success or a super fit body. Rather than cheating, find healthy foods that are your very favorites, and if you need to, splurge on something you really like that tastes great but is also healthy for you. I use fruits for this occasion, especially fruits I haven't had in a while or don't eat regularly so it still feels like something special. Give mangos a try. Does it get any better than that? Likely, but mangos make a strong case for being the ultimate tasty "cheat food" healthy substitute.

In addition to a no-junk-food diet plan and reduction in overall calories, you'll also want to create a fitness program that supports your nutritional efforts to drop body fat and improve muscle tone. A combination of weight training and cardiovascular or aerobic exercise will be mandatory. You need to train muscles to get them to stand out as well as put in the time with endurance training to burn calories and burn fat throughout your entire body.

When I think about toning up and burning fat, there are always specific types of athletes who come to mind, namely soccer players and basketball players. The athletes that play these sports have incredible muscle definition and tone, are ripped, cut, shredded, and have low levels of body fat. They do this by supporting their nutrition programs with amazing amounts of aerobic exercise. I think professional basketball players have some of the best physiques on the planet. Look no further than LeBron James and Dwight Howard, two of the most famous and successful players in the NBA, to see what running up and down a basketball court daily combined with periodic or regular weight training can do. Exercise contributes more to both muscle and bone strength and overall health than any supplement on the market.

When you get yourself into a good fat-burning fitness routine, you'll want to eat healthy plant-based whole foods to support all your athletic efforts. Both components—proper diet and exercise—work to support the other in a harmonious, synergistic relationship that will produce outstanding results. You can diet all you want and cut out all processed and refined foods and still not get muscle tone. You will just end up skinny. At first glance, sometimes it seems like basketball players and soccer players can get ripped no matter what diet they follow simply because of their intense exercise schedules, and it may seem that the nutrition aspect isn't that important. The truth is that nutrition is a huge key in their ability to maintain a lean and efficient physique. Every professional sports team in America has some sort of nutrition coach on staff to ensure athletes are following the fundamental principles involved in nutrition-related wellness. Nutrition plays a major role in our lives now and in the sustainability of our health in the future. Intense exercise is an exceptional way to tone-up the body, and a sound nutrition program supports it fully. The combination is superior to just one aspect alone.

One amusing thing is when women tell me they want to tone up but are afraid to lift weights because they don't want to get "too bulky." I just smile and then reply by telling them that I have dedicated my life to trying to get "bulky" with all the enthusiasm in the world and more testosterone and dedication than they have and still struggle to add bulk to my body. Bulking up is extremely hard to do unless you have amazing genetics or have put in many years of consistent training. Furthermore, men have an easier time because they have higher testosterone levels and are generally larger. I tell women there is nothing to be afraid of. Even with a toning fitness program of regular exercise using weights and aerobic training coupled with a toning nutrition program packed full of plant-based whole foods, it will still be hard to add a lot of bulk to the body. Rather the body will tone up nicely, meeting the goals set forth. Learn from the basketball players, soccer players, and other athletes with phenomenal physiques who display the kind of training and dedication required to support their nutrition program to achieve their goals.

Fat Burning Nutrition Programs

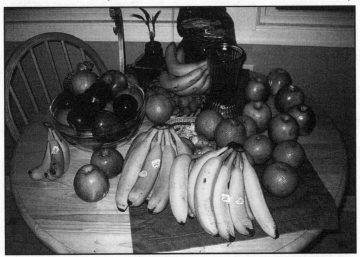

Photo by Robert Cheeke

Fat Burning Nutrition Program 1

Meal #1
3 pieces of whole fruit
Small bowl of oats
12 ounces of fresh squeezed juice
12 ounces of water

Meal #2
Assortment of mixed berries
Green protein drink
12 ounces of water

Meal #3
Large green salad with bean sprouts, cucumber, spinach,
    greens, and Vega omega 3-6-9 EFA oil
Vega meal replacement drink
12 ounces of water

Meal #4
3 pieces of whole fruit
2 Tablespoons of almond butter
Green smoothie
12 ounces of water

Meal #5
Large green salad with beans, broccoli, seaweed, other greens,
    and Vega omega 3-6-9 EFA oil
An assortment of nuts and seeds
12 ounces of water

Meal #6
2 pieces of whole fruit
Protein drink

Estimated Totals:
Total Calories = 3,500
Total grams protein = 165g
Total grams of carbohydrates = 500g
Total grams of fats = 100g
Total water consumption = 100 ounces (factoring in water for
    protein drinks too)

Fat Burning Nutrition Program 2

Meal #1
   3 pieces of exotic fruit
   3 ounces of wheatgrass
   Green smoothie with protein powder
   12 ounces of water

Meal #2
   Assortment of vegetables with hummus or bean dip
   12 ounce natural vitamin drink or pre-workout drink
   12 ounces of water

Meal #3
   Bowl of quinoa with greens and tempeh
   Small green salad
   12 ounces of water

Meal #4
   3 pieces of whole fruit
   Flax crackers with almond butter
   Green smoothie with Vega Smoothie Infusion
   12 ounces of water

Meal #5
   Yam fries with dark leafy green vegetables and Vega omega
       3-6-9 EFA oil
   Bowl of asparagus and broccoli
   Small salad with hemp seeds and pumpkin seeds
   12 ounces of water

Meal #6
   3 pieces of whole fruit
   Vega meal replacement drink
   12 ounces of water

Estimated Totals:
   Total Calories = 4,000
   Total grams protein = 190g
   Total grams of carbohydrates = 600g
   Total grams of fats = 90g
   Total water consumption = 108 ounces (factoring in water for
       protein drinks too)

Fat Burning Nutrition Program 3

Meal #1
5 rice cakes with almond butter
Bowl of oats with Vega meal replacement powder mixed in
2 pieces of whole fruit chopped up and put in oats
12 ounces of water

Meal #2
Dates and coconut flakes
Green Smoothie with Vega Smoothie Infusion
2 pieces of whole fruit
12 ounces of water

Meal #3
2 yams with almond gravy or peanut sauce
Strips of tempeh with kale salad
12 ounces of hemp milk
Sun Warrior rice protein drink
12 ounces of water

Meal #4
Large green salad with lots of veggies, beans, peas, and a
    variety of greens
Kombucha drink
Vega meal replacement drink
12 ounces of water

Meal #5
Stir fried vegetables with tofu or steamed vegetables with tofu
Small green salad with Vega omega 3-6-9 EFA oil and hemp
    seeds
12 ounces of water

Meal #6
Protein drink or protein smoothie
2 pieces of whole fruit
12 ounces of water

Estimated Totals:
Total Calories = 4,500
Total grams protein = 225g
Total grams of carbohydrates = 675g
Total grams of fats = 100g
Total water consumption = 120 ounces (factoring in water for
protein drinks too)

Though some of the nutrition totals may seem high for fat burning, keep in mind many people burn 4,500 calories a day just in daily life activities such as walking, commuting, exercising, and sexual activity. Additionally, there is a high amount of essential fats in my suggestions. The consumption of essential fats helps burn fat and speeds up the metabolism making fat burning more efficient.

Pre-Contest Nutrition Program

The Pre-Contest nutrition program is the most complicated and perhaps the most crucial in the entire bodybuilding season. This is where all the cards are on the table, everything is on the line, and you find out what you're made of. This is where some people can't handle the restrictions or specifics that

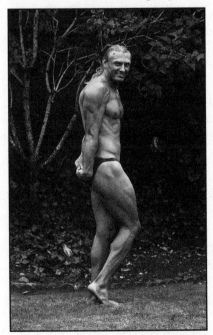

are part of the nutrition program during this period of time, and this is where others thrive and leave their mark on the sport. It is by far the most challenging time of the year for a bodybuilder. The goal is to be in the best possible shape on a specific day. Bodybuilders allow themselves anywhere from 12-16 weeks to create and follow a detailed plan to drop body fat and get ripped, while maintaining hard-earned muscle before getting on stage. During this 12-16 week period, bodybuilders manipulate many aspects of their diet from carbohydrate, fat, and protein consumption to sodium and water intake. They increase cardiovascular training up to two or three hours a day and often reduce carbohydrate in-

Photo by Randall Perez –
RandallPerez.com

take, leaving barely enough energy to get through the workouts. This is the aspect of bodybuilding that challenges me the most each and every time I compete. Sometimes I handle the pre-contest diet well; other times it has gotten the best of me, and I have given in and have succumbed to less than desirable results and have been forced to make excuses or admit my shortcomings and make new commitments for future competitions. Whether I am successful or unsuccessful in sticking with the outlined diet, there is always a lesson learned and room for improvement discovered.

The pre-contest diet period is truly the time when your character traits come out the most. It is when your frustration is revealed and also when your warrior-like mentality comes through and you display that you are tougher and more committed than most give you credit for. It is when you find out exactly how weak you really are and when you discover how strong you really are. It is during this time when you realize that your heart is the strongest muscle in your body no matter how big or small your physique is. This is the time when some say, "I can't take it anymore," and when others say, "Yes, I can do this." It is such as a wonderful opportunity to learn so much about yourself. I wish everyone could experience bodybuilding for themselves just for this rare opportunity to have a three-month period of self talk, constantly battling with your own mind, questioning what you're made of, and revealing aspects about your human character you never knew before. It's the part of bodybuilding that makes you never want to do it again and the same part of bodybuilding that nearly makes you addicted to it, creating a desire to improve upon your prior self and compete year after year.

The whole idea around the pre-contest diet is to do all the fat burning and physique altering modifications that need to be made to get you stage-ready for competition. The reason bodybuilders don't follow a pre-contest diet year-round is because it is challenging and very hard to maintain. They eat specific foods, often a fairly limited diet, increase workouts, and demand more from themselves. Bodybuilders use the off-season to add overall mass, weight, and a bit of body fat which allows them to be heavier and bigger and capable of becoming stronger which helps build muscle. Bodybuilders build mass for most of the year and then dedicate a three-month period to toning up, getting shredded and contest stage-ready. The goal is to hang onto the muscle put on during the six to nine months mass building and just strip away the body fat pre-contest. Some mix in a maintenance diet as well. There is a bulking phase, a maintaining phase, a toning phase, and then a contest-ready ripping up phase just prior to competition. Some bodybuilders use a maintenance phase year-round and don't worry about bulking up with extra body fat but prefer to stay lean all throughout the year. Others do dramatic transformations from a big increase in body fat to significant drops in body fat in the final few months before competition. Others yet will spend only four to eight weeks for their pre-contest diet and training programs while others spend 16-20 weeks on a specific nutrition program designed to get them ready to be on stage in their best condition possible. We all have our own strategies, and of course, I have my own preferences as well.

I adopt a pre-contest diet 12 weeks away from a bodybuilding competition. That diet evolves throughout that three-month time frame. With 12 weeks before the competition, I start eliminating junk foods, cut down on refined and processed foods, and focus more on whole foods as much as possible. After about a month of eating more fresh foods and less processed foods, with about eight weeks to go before being on stage, I again evaluate my diet and remove all breads, pastas, and other processed foods that are high in carbohydrates and which are not whole foods. I also increase my protein intake so my carbohydrate intake will diminish naturally. At this juncture, I also increase my cardiovascular training and become a little more cautious with my training to prevent injuries, as I'm only two months from being on stage. As I lower carbohydrate consumption (main source for fuel or energy), I make an extra effort to be careful in the gym knowing I don't have quite as much energy.

With about six weeks before the competition, I'll often reduce high sugar content foods, including natural sources like fruits. I cut down my overall consumption of fruits, sometimes completely eliminate energy bars, and I really put an emphasis on high protein foods, green foods, low sodium foods, and I keep my fluid intake high. For a recent competition I didn't eat a single energy bar for six whole weeks! I normally eat at least one a day, and sometimes three or four a day, so it was an interesting experience to remove a staple food that is also a convenience food from my diet for that length of time.

A month before the competition, I try to step it up a notch in every area from the foods I'm eating to the rest I'm getting, to the intensity and dedication of my training programs. I train longer if I feel like I need to burn more fat. I spend more time practicing posing so I can see how my body looks and evaluate changes I need to make. I make sure my diet is really clean focusing on high protein foods, low carbohydrate foods, and good supplementation to keep my energy levels up and immune system strong.

When I am just 14 days away from the competition, I will drop my carbohydrate intake to about 50 grams a day for 10-12 days and then carbohydrate-load about 36-48 hours before getting on stage. I do this to shock the body to some degree and deprive it of carbohydrates so I can burn fat rather than store fat and get leaner as a result. Then I will pump my muscles full of carbohydrates just before the competition to make the muscles full again—packed full of energy. The carbohydrates actually re-shape the muscles, making each one appear bigger and more full and rounded.

When I'm closing in on the competition date, I also cut out my use of the supplement creatine, which by its nature retains water in the body—something I certainly don't want when on the bodybuilding stage. I want the look of a very dry and hard body revealing details in every muscle. I cut out creatine weeks before the competition, but I continue my use of the muscle-building amino acid L-glutamine to help with muscle recovery and immune system support. Recently, my posing coach Andre Scott advised me to discontinue use of protein drinks in the final days leading up to the competition because some of the sweeteners could have an impact on how my body looks and because the use of protein drinks often includes water. If I do consume protein drinks just before a competition, I make sure to use only enough water with the powder to get it to mix from a powder to more of a pudding or thick shake. The water I do ingest is distilled with the sodium and minerals removed, and I tend to drink small quantities, getting enough to keep my body functioning properly but not enough to make my body look soft.

The pre-contest diet meal programs I am going to list are the types of programs you would find me following two to four weeks away from competition. My diet gets a little crazy during the final couple of days before contest, and I'll describe what that is like as well and list a couple of samples of what my nutritional consumption would be. But the following represent what may be expected from me with about half a month to a month from competition.

Pre-Contest Bodybuilding Meal Programs

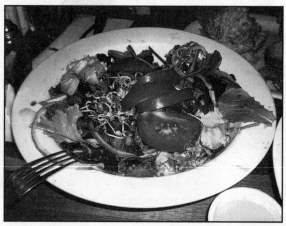

Photo by Robert Cheeke

Pre-Contest Meal Program #1

Meal #1

    Large bowl of oatmeal with a scoop of Vega meal replacement
       powder
    16 ounce green protein drink
    12 ounces of distilled water

Meal #2

    Sun Warrior rice protein drink
    2 rice cakes with almond butter
    12 ounces of distilled water

Meal #3

    Large green salad with tofu, a variety of greens and other
       veggies, and Vega omega 3-6-9 EFA oil
    1-2 servings of walnuts
    12 ounces of distilled water

Meal #4

    Sun Warrior rice protein drink
    2 rice cakes with almond butter
    12 ounces of distilled water

Meal #5

    Vega Sport pre-workout drink
    Nitric Oxide drink
    1 orange

Meal #6

    1 bowl of quinoa with kale and tempeh
    Vega Sport Protein with BCAA's and L-glutamine included
    12 ounces of distilled water

Meal #7

    Sun Warrior rice protein drink
    Zero/low carbohydrate organic tofu with greens and Vega omega
       3-6-9 EFA oil
    Multi vitamin and other vitamin supplements
    12 ounces of distilled water

Estimated Totals:
Total Calories = 3,200
Total grams protein = 250g
Total grams of carbohydrates = 260g
Total grams of fats = 130g
Total water consumption = 168 ounces (factoring in water for
    protein drinks too)

Pre-Contest Meal Program #2

Meal #1
Vega/Sun Warrior protein drink
2 pieces of sprouted grain bread with almond butter
Handful of blueberries
12 ounces of distilled water

Meal #2
2 servings of almonds
2 servings of walnuts
2 rice cakes with coconut oil
12 ounces of distilled water

Meal #3
Bowl of baked tofu with nutritional yeast
½ yam
1 cup of broccoli
12 ounces of distilled water

Meal #4
Sun Warrior rice protein drink
2 slices of sprouted bread with mung beans and avocado
12 ounces of distilled water
Vega Sport pre-workout drink

Meal #5
Bowl of brown rice with kidney beans, garbanzo beans, an assortment of greens, and hummus
VEGA Sport Protein drink with BCAA's and L-glutamine included
12 ounces of distilled water

Meal #6
Bowl of quinoa with baked tofu and greens with Vega omega
3-6-9 EFA oil
Pure Advantage pea protein drink with amino acid L-glutamine
12 ounces of distilled water

Meal #7
Sun warrior rice protein drink
2 rice cakes with almond butter
12 ounces of distilled water

Estimated Totals:
Total Calories = 4,000
Total grams protein = 250g
Total grams of carbohydrates = 400g
Total grams of fats = 150g
Total water consumption = 144 ounces (factoring in water for
protein drinks too)

Pre-Contest Meal Program #3

Meal #1
Sun Warrior rice protein drink with L-glutamine
12 ounces of distilled water

Meal #2
Baked tofu and spinach
Vega meal replacement drink
12 ounces of distilled water

Meal #3
Sun Warrior rice protein drink with L-glutamine
Baked tofu with green salad and Vega omega 3-6-9 EFA oil
12 ounces of distilled water

Meal #4
Protein drink
3 rice cakes and almond butter
12 ounces of distilled water

Meal #5
Steamed broccoli and other vegetables with tempeh
Seaweed salad
Protein drink
12 ounces of distilled water

Meal #6
Vega Sport Protein drink with BCAA's and L-glutamine included
Small green salad
12 ounces of water

Meal #7
4 rice cakes with almond butter
12 ounces of water

Estimated Totals:
Total Calories = 3,000
Total grams protein = 250g
Total grams of carbohydrates = 320g
Total grams of fats = 80g
Total water consumption = 156 ounces (factoring in water for protein drinks too)

Carbohydrate-load Pre-Contest meal plan for Final 2 Days Before Competition

Two days before contest Meal Program #1

Meal #1
10 rice cakes with almond butter on 4 of them
1 bowl of oatmeal
Vega Smoothie Infusion with frozen fruit
12 ounces of water

Meal #2
4 slices of sprouted bread with almond butter
Sun Warrior rice protein drink
12 ounces of water

Meal #3

Bowl of brown rice with veggies, greens, and organic unflavored
tofu
Vega meal replacement drink

Meal #4

1 yam with greens and Vega omega 3-6-9 EFA oil
Sun Warrior rice protein drink

Meal #5

1 yam with greens
Sun Warrior rice protein drink

Meal #6

1 yam
Baked unflavored tofu with greens and Vega omega 3-6-9
EFA oil

Meal #7

5 rice cakes with almond butter

Estimated Totals:

Total Calories = 3,500
Total grams protein = 240g
Total grams of carbohydrates = 465g
Total grams of fats = 75g
Total water consumption = 84 ounces (factoring in water for
protein drinks too)

Two days before the competition Meal Program #2

Meal #1

Bowl of oatmeal with Vega meal replacement powder
Green protein smoothie
8 ounces of water

Meal #2

Sun Warrior Protein drink
1 grapefruit

Meal #3
1 yam
Baked tofu with small green salad
Vega Sport Protein drink with BCAA's and L-glutamine included

Meal #4
Vega meal replacement drink
Small bowl of asparagus

Meal #5
6 rice cakes with almond butter
Vega Sport Protein drink with BCAA's and L-glutamine included

Meal #6
Sun Warrior rice protein drink
1 grapefruit

Meal #7
4 slices of sprouted bread with almond butter
Vitamins/digestive enzymes

Estimated Totals:
Total Calories = 3,000
Total grams protein = 230g
Total grams of carbohydrates = 390g
Total grams of fats = 60g
Total water consumption = 80 ounces (factoring in water for
    protein drinks too)

Day before competition Meal Programs

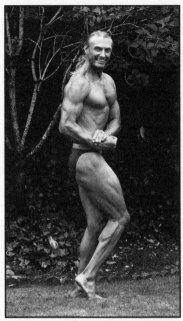

*Photo by Randall Perez –
RandallPerez.com*

Day before competition
Meal Program #1

Meal #1
Bowl of oatmeal
7 rice cakes, 3 of them with almond butter

Meal #2
½ yam with bowl of greens

Meal #3
1 cup brown rice with unflavored baked
    tofu
Sun Warrior rice protein drink

Meal #4
½ yam and unflavored baked tofu

Meal #5
    ½ yam with bowl of greens
    Vega meal replacement drink

Meal #6
    Bowl of brown rice with baked tofu and greens

Meal #7
    ½ yam
    3 rice cakes with almond butter

Estimated Totals:
    Total Calories = 2,800
    Total grams protein = 190g
    Total grams of carbohydrates = 400g
    Total grams of fats = 50g
    Total water consumption = 24 ounces (factoring in water for
        protein drinks too)

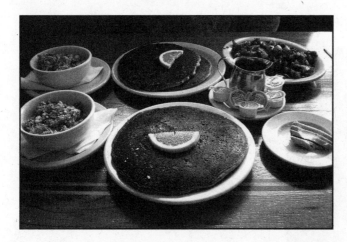

*Vegan Pancakes from
Cup and Saucer in
Portland, OR*

Day before competition Meal Program #2

Meal #1
> 3 large pancakes with maple syrup
> Small cup of assorted berries or other fruit
> Vega Sport Protein drink with BCAA's and L-glutamine included

Meal #2
> 5 rice cakes with almond butter
> 2 carrots with almond butter

Meal #3
> Large plate of pasta with low sodium peanut sauce or almond
>   butter
> Green salad with Vega omega 3-6-9 EFA oil
> 1 English cucumber

Meal #4
> Vega meal replacement drink
> 5 rice cakes with almond butter

Meal #5
> Dish with tofu, mixed vegetables, and noodles
> Green salad with Vega omega 3-6-9 EFA oil

Meal #6
> Bowl of quinoa with kale and tempeh
> 1 grapefruit

Estimated Totals:
Total Calories = 4,800
Total grams protein = 240g
Total grams of carbohydrates = 665g
Total grams of fats = 130g
Total water consumption = 24 ounces (factoring in water for protein drinks too)

Day of competition Meal Programs

Day of Competition Meal Program #1

Meal #1
(early in the morning, hours before pre-judging)
10 rice cakes
12 ounce Vega Sport pre-work-out drink
1 chocolate bar

Meal #2
(two hours before getting on stage)
1 cup sliced yams (prepared the day before)
12 ounce Vega Sport pre-work-out drink

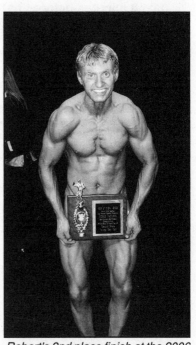

Meal #3
(15-30 minutes before getting on stage, to be eaten while pumping up)

Robert's 2nd place finish at the 2006 INBA Natural Bodybuilding World Championships

1 orange
Handful of candy or high sugar food
Part of a chocolate bar

Meal #4
(immediately after getting off stage)
32 ounces of water
1 cup of sliced yams
Vega meal replacement drink

Meal #5
(lunch)

Eat whatever you feel like. All decisions are made during pre-judging unless you win your class and compete for the overall title. If you are fighting for an overall title, keep lunch small to avoid bloating and continue to eat high carbohydrate foods such as yams, rice cakes, almond butter, and fruit.

Meal #6
(30-60 minutes before finals)

12 ounce Vega Sport pre-workout drink
½ chocolate bar
16 ounces of water

Meal #7
(post competition immediately after getting off stage)

Any snack or meal you have been craving for weeks or months. Enjoy yourself; you're done for the evening.
32 ounces of water

Meal #8
(Dinner)

Eat whatever you'd like for dinner. You've earned it

Estimated Totals:

Total Calories = Varies based on your lunch and dinner meals of choice

Total grams protein = Varies based on your lunch and dinner meals of choice

Total grams of carbohydrates = Varies based on your lunch and dinner meals of choice

Total grams of fats = Varies based on your lunch and dinner meals of choice

Total water consumption = Varies based on your lunch and dinner meals of choice

Day of Competition Meal Program #2

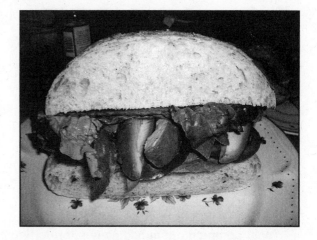

*Avocado sandwich
made by Julia Abbott*

Meal #1
(early in the morning, hours before pre-judging)
>   4 pancakes with maple syrup
>   Tofu sausage or other protein source for breakfast
>   2 grapefruits
>   16 ounce orange juice

Meal #2
(two hours before getting on stage)
>   6 small red potatoes
>   English cucumber dipped in almond butter
>   12 ounce Vega Sport pre-workout drink

Meal #3
(15-30 minutes before getting on stage, to be eaten while pumping up)
>   1 grapefruit
>   1 chocolate bar and other candies
>   8 ounce Vega Sport pre-workout drink

Meal #4
(immediately after getting off stage)
>   5 rice cakes with almond butter
>   3 red potatoes
>   1 grapefruit
>   16 ounce Vega Sport pre-workout drink

Meal #5
(lunch)

Eat whatever you feel like. All decisions are made during pre-judging unless you win your class and compete for the overall title. If you are fighting for an overall title, keep lunch small to avoid bloating and continue to eat high carbohydrate foods such as yams, rice cakes, almond butter, and fruit.

Meal #6
(30-60 minutes before finals)

1 grapefruit
Half of a chocolate bar and other candies
12 ounce Vega Sport pre-workout drink

Meal #7
(post competition immediately after getting off stage)

Any snack or meal you have been craving for weeks or months. Enjoy yourself; you're done for the evening.
32 ounces of water

Meal #8
(Dinner)

Eat whatever you'd like for dinner. You've earned it

Estimated Totals:

Total Calories = Varies based on your lunch and dinner
    meals of choice
Total grams protein = Varies based on your lunch and
    dinner meals of choice
Total grams of carbohydrates = Varies based on your lunch
    and dinner meals of choice
Total grams of fats = Varies based on your lunch and
    dinner meals of choice
Total water consumption = Varies based on your lunch and
    dinner meals of choice

Maintenance Nutrition Program

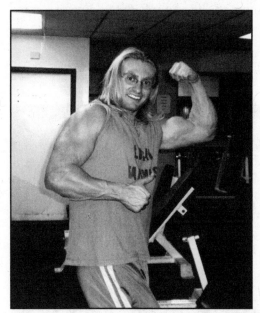

Photo by Javier de la Camara

Maintaining what you've worked hard to achieve should be a goal of yours and easy to attain. Improvement can be challenging depending on the vision, but simply maintaining a certain physique throughout the year is quite easy for many. The only time this really becomes challenging is when you make the decision not to train or eat sufficiently. Sometimes bodybuilders burn out from competitions and from intense training and dieting and take time off. Occasionally they take off more time than initially planned. It is during these times that bodybuilders don't give themselves the appropriate opportunities to even maintain weight or maintain their bodybuilding physiques. Numerous times throughout my life I have taken breaks from bodybuilding for one reason or another, and each and every time I found it hard to maintain what I had worked so hard to build. It was frustrating each and every time because years of bodybuilding training can be washed away in weeks of not training or eating like a bodybuilder. I have suffered through a case of mononucleosis only weeks before a scheduled competition, multiple major back injuries, and other injuries or setbacks so I have had lots of experience with the feeling of starting over, even after impressive gains I worked hard to achieve.

To maintain our physiques efficiently, we must understand the importance of the maintenance period of our bodybuilding lifestyle. Just because we don't have a competition coming up doesn't mean we should stop living the bodybuilding lifestyle. To maintain muscle and avoid catabolic experiences, our maintenance nutrition program becomes imperative for continued success. The great thing about this period of time for bodybuilders is that we can typically eat whatever we want without having various restrictions in our diet, live without the mood swings that come along with dieting, and go about our day without having it become a chore to take in supplements or specific nutrient proportions at exact times. We can simply eat our favorite foods, keep our meal frequency up, continue on with our training, and keep progressing until we're ready for the next period of our bodybuilding program.

The maintenance meal programs include six meals a day which is most common and highly attainable.

Maintenance Meal Programs

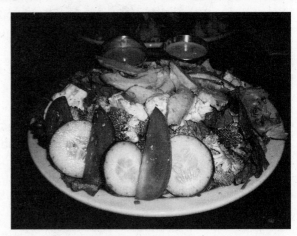

Large salad from Nearly Normals Vegetarian Restaurant – Corvallis, OR

Maintenance Meal Program #1

Meal #1
Bowl of oatmeal
Green protein smoothie
2 pieces of whole fruit
16 ounces of water

Meal #2
2 protein or energy bars
1 cucumber
1 carrot
16 ounces of water

Meal #3
Large green salad with mixed greens and Vega omega 3-6-9
EFA oil
2 artichokes and bowl of mixed beans and sprouts
Protein drink
16 ounces of water

Meal #4
Celery sticks with almond butter
2 pieces of whole fruit
16 ounces of water

Meal #5
Ethiopian food dinner (bread and beans, greens, lentils,
hummus, and a variety of other dips)
16 ounces of water

Meal #6
Tofu "chicken" sandwich with vegan mayonnaise, lettuce, and
tomato
Bowl of rice with peanut sauce and green side salad
16 ounces of water

Estimated Totals:
Total Calories = 4300
Total grams protein = 175g
Total grams of carbohydrates = 675g
Total grams of fats = 100g
Total water consumption = 120 ounces (factoring in water for
protein drinks too)

Maintenance Meal Program #2

Meal #1
2 pieces of whole fruit
Yerba maté drink
Fruit Smoothie

Meal #2
Energy bar
Assorted fresh vegetables (carrots, cucumbers, peppers)
16 ounces of water

Meal #3
Burrito with rice or quinoa, greens, beans, and avocado
Small green salad with Vega omega 3-6-9 EFA oil
12 ounces of hemp milk
16 ounces of water

Meal #4
>   2 pieces of whole fruit
>   Protein drink
>   16 ounces of water

Meal #5
>   Large green salad with steamed green vegetables and tempeh
>   Bowl of carrot/ginger soup
>   12 ounces of almond milk
>   16 ounces of water

Meal #6
>   Protein bar
>   Protein drink
>   1 piece of fruit
>   16 ounces of water

Estimated Totals:
>   Total Calories = 4,000
>   Total grams protein = 180g
>   Total grams of carbohydrates = 660g
>   Total grams of fats = 70g
>   Total water consumption = 104 ounces (factoring in water for
>   protein drinks too)

Maintenance Meal Program #3

Meal #1
>   2 pancakes with maple syrup
>   Small bowl of potatoes and broccoli
>   16 ounces of fresh squeezed orange juice
>   16 ounces of water

Meal #2
>   Almond butter sandwich with jam
>   Green protein smoothie
>   16 ounces of water

Meal #3
Collard green wraps with hummus or vegetable pate, beans,
    sprouts, and vegetables
Bowl of lentil, bean, or vegetable soup
16 ounces of water

Meal #4
3 pieces of whole fruit
An assortment of nuts (2-3 servings)
16 ounces of water

Meal #5
Bell peppers stuffed with rice and seasonings
Green salad with Vega omega 3-6-9 EFA oil
Bean sprouts and fresh or steamed vegetables
16 ounces of water

Meal #6
Vega meal replacement drink
2 pieces of whole fruit

Estimated Totals:
Total Calories = 4,500
Total grams protein = 160g
Total grams of carbohydrates = 760g
Total grams of fats = 90g
Total water consumption = 104 ounces (factoring in water for
    protein drinks too)

Raw Food Vegan Bodybuilding

I have to admit, I didn't think it could be done. I didn't think bodybuild-ing on a 100% raw food diet was possible with any sort of real effectiveness until I met Raw Food Vegan Bodybuilder Giacomo Marchese in the summer of 2008. Giacomo attended a summer gathering for Vegan Bodybuilding & Fitness (www.veganbodybuilding.com) members in Portland, OR, and it was during that vacation that I saw for the first time a raw foodist who didn't look undernourished. Rather, he looked very strong and was very strong. Giacomo completely changed the way I viewed raw foods as a diet and lifestyle pro-gram, or at least uniquely changed the way I viewed the raw food lifestyle as he lived it. The raw food diet doesn't interest me, but my friend Giacomo not

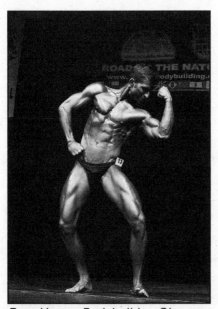

Raw Vegan Bodybuilder Giacomo Marchese – (photo by Randall Perez – RandallPerez.com)

only lives it but also combines it with bodybuilding—an incredibly tough endeavor. Giacomo has the ability to hone in on a specific goal and work exceptionally hard to achieve it. He does what most aren't willing to do, and he achieves uncommon results because of that approach. Like any other diet or nutritional lifestyle choice, bodybuilding on 100% raw foods should be done properly for efficient results and positive overall health.

After two weeks of visiting Portland, OR for our Vegan Vacation 2008, Giacomo returned home to Brooklyn, NY and then only months later moved to Portland, OR with his girlfriend Dani whom he met during our Vegan Vacation. Giacomo and I became better friends and started training together. I learned more about the raw food vegan bodybuilding lifestyle directly as a result of observation and time spent with him. In late 2008, I approached Giacomo asking if he wanted to participate in my documentary *Vegan Brothers in Iron*. The documentary would be about our lives as vegan bodybuilders, and the cameras would follow us for 12 weeks as we trained, ate, and lived the vegan bodybuilding lifestyle. Giacomo enthusiastically agreed, and I recruited Producer Brian Van Peski to help us make it a reality. Our vegan bodybuilding friend Jimi Sitko later joined the team, and we set out to impact audiences in a project that fully engulfed and encompassed our lives for more than three months.

When I first asked Giacomo to be part of the *Vegan Brothers in Iron* documentary, I questioned my own decision to invite him because of his raw food diet and the controversy around that lifestyle, especially as it related to bodybuilding. I also questioned his involvement because at the time I approached him, he was very stressed out as a result of his recent cross-country move and was skinnier than normal. I wasn't sure what kind of representative he would be for the vegan bodybuilding lifestyle. He had just moved 3,000 miles from home and was looking for a job and trying to get settled in his new community; going to the gym wasn't high on his priority list, rather making friends, finding employment, and acquainting himself with his new town were. When he accepted my invitation to be part of the documentary, he got right to work in the gym and in the kitchen. On a 100% raw food diet he went from his tired and stressed-out physique of 167 pounds to a ripped, strong, and solid 187 pounds in about three weeks! Yes, in just three weeks, all on raw foods! He accomplished this by doing things that most people I know aren't willing to do, which is why he stands out and why he is exceptional. He ate pounds of sprouted mung beans everyday and drank a gallon or more of algae or other green drinks on a daily basis. He consumed loads of protein and calories, and his body responded well. He spent hours in the gym lifting heavy weights, even with an injured shoulder and amidst continued stress in his life. He rose to the occasion and shocked many people around him with his transformation in such a short time and on a 100% raw food diet. He became incredibly strong; his muscles were large and hard, and I was inspired by his results. I wasn't inspired to eat a raw food diet and wasn't inspired to explore the raw food lifestyle more, but I was inspired by his dedication, his consistency, his passion, and his ability to overcome obstacles in his life. I was also inspired by his commitment to me and our documentary project. He truly inspired a lot of people around him and gave many of us pause as we saw something we had never seen before, an exceptionally strong and muscular person in the raw food community. I honestly believe that when Giacomo embraces the opportunities he'll create for himself, he will be the next big thing in the raw food movement. It is only a matter of time until he takes his raw vegan bodybuilding career to the next level.

Through my observations as a co-producer and co-star of *Vegan Brothers in Iron*, I've seen what can result with extreme commitment and dedication that is fueled by the desire to improve and excel. I've now learned that it IS possible to be a 100% raw food vegan bodybuilder, and Giacomo is a testament to that and a shining example. Giacomo is bound to emerge as a leader in the raw food movement in the very near future.

I admire and applaud Giacomo for the example he is setting. He is much like my friend John Kohler, who has been a raw foodist for the past 12 years. They both focus on food as their primary source of nutrition rather than magical products, extracts, and expensive raw food supplements. Simply, they eat real, fresh plant-based whole foods in raw, uncooked forms. They are both fantastic role models for people interested in eating a healthy raw food diet. I believe they eat the way the raw food diet was intended: consumption of real food that comes from the ground, a tree, or bush rather than dried, packaged extracts that are mostly tools for making money and building reputations. Giacomo and John go back to the basics and grow their own food in gardens. They eat a healthy variety of fresh foods and thrive on their 100% raw food diets and seem to truly enjoy themselves and enjoy life. That is the kind of role model I really look up to.

From my observations and conversations and videotaped sessions with Giacomo, coupled with my own ideas, I've come up with some raw food bodybuilding meal programs.

For more information about raw food vegan bodybuilding, check out www.veganproteins.com and get in touch with Giacomo Marchese. I believe he is the best ambassador for raw food vegan bodybuilding today. He is irresistibly outgoing, caring, and helpful. I know that he would be happy to hear from you. Find him on his website or on Facebook or @VeganProteins on Twitter. Tell him "RC" sent you. You can also search John Kohler online and use him as a solid role model in the raw food movement.

Raw Food Bodybuilding Meal Programs

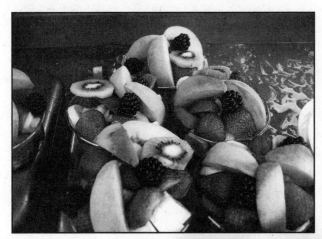

*Photos by
Robert Cheeke*

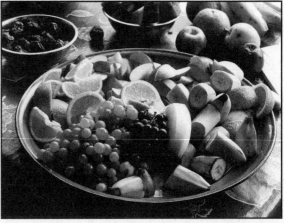

Raw Food Bodybuilding Meal Program #1

Meal #1
32 ounce spirulina protein drink
Sun Warrior rice protein drink
2 pieces of whole fruit
16 ounces of water

Meal #2
Large bowl of sprouted mung beans with cayenne pepper
16 ounce spirulina protein drink
Sun Warrior rice protein drink
16 ounces of water

Meal #3
Large green salad with lots of dark greens, seeds, and bean
    sprouts with Vega omega 3-6-9 EFA oil
16 ounce spirulina protein drink
16 ounces of water

Meal #4
Large bowl of mung bean sprouts with herbs or seasoning
Sun Warrior rice protein drink
16 ounces of water

Meal #5
16 ounce spirulina protein drink
Large green salad with sprouts, vegetables, and seeds
16 ounces of water

Meal #6
Sun Warrior rice protein drink
Bowl of sprouts
16 ounces of water

Estimated Totals:
Total Calories = 3,000
Total grams protein = 250g
Total grams of carbohydrates = 430g
Total grams of fats = 30g
Total water consumption = 224 ounces (factoring in water for
    protein drinks too)

Raw Food Bodybuilding Meal Program #2

Meal #1
3 pieces of whole fruit
24 ounce spirulina protein drink
Sun Warrior rice protein drink
16 ounces of water

Meal #2
3 servings of whole fruit
16 ounce spirulina protein drink
Sun Warrior rice protein drink
16 ounces of water

Meal #3
Large green salad with lots of sprouts
Sun Warrior rice protein drink
16 ounces of water

Meal #4
2 raw energy bars
16 ounce kombucha tea
16 ounces of water

Meal #5
16 ounce spirulina protein drink
Large zucchini pasta salad with greens, sprouts, and raw oils
16 ounces of water

Meal #6
2 servings of raw nuts
Green salad
Sun Warrior rice protein drink

Estimated Totals:
Total Calories = 3,500
Total grams protein = 200g
Total grams of carbohydrates = 585g
Total grams of fats = 40g
Total water consumption = 192 ounces (factoring water for
protein drinks too)

Raw Food Bodybuilding Meal Program #3

Meal #1
> 3 pieces of whole fruit
> 2 raw food energy bars
> Green smoothie
> 16 ounces of water

Meal #2
> 2 servings of dates with coconut flakes
> 2 servings of durian
> 16 ounce spirulina protein drink
> 16 ounces of water

Meal #3
> Large green salad with bean sprouts, kale, seaweed, and other
> greens
> 2 cucumbers
> Green smoothie
> 16 ounces of water

Meal #4
> Sun Warrior rice protein drink
> 2 raw food bars
> 2 servings of raw nuts
> 2 pieces of whole fruit
> 16 ounces of water

Meal #5
> Large bowl of sprouted mung beans
> Flax crackers with raw hummus
> Carrots, cucumber, and artichoke hearts with green salad
> 16 ounces of water

Meal #6
> Sun Warrior rice protein drink
> Kale salad
> Green smoothie

Estimated Totals:
Total Calories = 5,200
Total grams protein = 230g
Total grams of carbohydrates = 845g
Total grams of fats = 100g
Total water consumption = 170 ounces (factoring in water for
protein drinks too)

Soy and Gluten-Free Vegan Bodybuilding Meal Programs

Since there are so
many people with aller-
gies, I wanted to present
a few meal programs free
of soy, gluten, and all
common allergens.

Of course, one of the
best ways to avoid com-
mon allergens is to eat
fresh plant-based whole
foods as often as pos-
sible—fruits, vegetables,
nuts, grains, and seeds. It

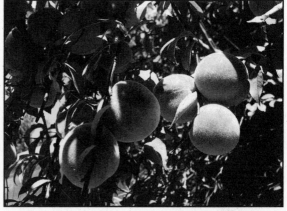

Photo by Robert Cheeke

is when foods are heavily processed that problems arise. Not all naturally
occurring foods are healthy, some are toxic or poisonous, but the vast majority of common plant-based whole foods are often our best bet for overall
health. Some foods like soybeans are toxic in their raw, natural state and
need to be processed to some degree before consumption. Not all "processed" foods are exceptionally bad for us, and I do enjoy a variety of them.
In general, the best way to get the best nutrition and to steer clear from common allergens is to avoid processed foods and eat whole foods.

These meal plans are intended to appeal to anyone and focus on whole
foods and other foods, supplements, and food bars that are free of common
allergens and additives.

Soy-Free and Gluten Free (all common allergen-free) Meal Programs

Common Allergen-free Meal Program #1

Meal #1
3 pieces of whole fruit
Vega meal replacement drink (all common allergen-free)
16 ounces of water

Meal #2
1 Vega bar (common allergy-free bar)
Assortment of fresh vegetables with hummus
Green smoothie
16 ounces of water

Meal #3
Large green salad with a variety of vegetables, seeds, and Vega
  omega 3-6-9 EFA oil
16 ounce kombucha tea
16 ounces of water

Meal #4
2 raw food bars
2 pieces of whole fruit
Sun Warrior rice protein drink
16 ounces of water

Meal #5
2 baked yams with steamed broccoli and other vegetables
Multi-bean salad with sprouts
Green smoothie

Meal #6
Flax crackers with cashew butter
Seaweed salad
16 ounce kombucha tea

Estimated Totals:
Total Calories = 4,300
Total grams protein = 190g
Total grams of carbohydrates = 680g
Total grams of fats = 90g
Total water consumption = 112 ounces (factoring in water for
  protein drinks too)

Common Allergen-free Meal Program #2

Meal #1
Bowl of common allergen-free cereal with Vega meal
    replacement powder
Sprouted common allergen-free bread with almond butter and jam
16 ounces of fresh squeezed juice

Meal #2
Vega bar
3 pieces of whole fruit
Sun Warrior rice protein drink
16 ounces of water

Meal #3
12 sushi rolls "sliced up from two full size rolls" (rice and
    seaweed with avocado and cucumber)
½ roasted squash with steamed vegetables
16 ounces of water

Meal #4
2 pieces of whole fruit
1 raw food bar
16 ounces of water

Meal #5
Bowl of quinoa with kale, spinach, and a variety of beans and sprouts
Small green salad with seeds and common allergen-free nuts
16 ounces of water

Meal #6
Sun Warrior rice protein drink
2 pieces of whole tropical fruit such as mangos, nectarines, or
dragon fruit
16 ounces of water

Estimated Totals:
Total Calories = 3,800
Total grams protein = 175g
Total grams of carbohydrates = 550g
Total grams of fats = 90g
Total water consumption = 104 ounces (factoring in water for
    protein drinks too)

Common Allergen-free Meal Program #3

Meal #1
Large fruit salad with a lot of variety of fresh fruits with sprouted
buckwheat (gluten-free)
Green smoothie
16 ounces of water

Meal #2
Dried fruit and mixed common allergen-free nuts and seeds in
trail mix
Vega meal replacement drink
16 ounces of water

Meal #3
Large green salad with walnuts and pecans
Collard green wrap with hummus and peppers
16 ounces of water

Meal #4
Vega bar
2 pieces of whole fruit
16 ounce kombucha tea

Meal #5
Bowl of brown rice with curry sauce and a variety of vegetables
Bowl of lentil/vegetable soup
16 ounce yerba maté
16 ounces of water

Meal #6
16 ounce spirulina protein drink
8 ounce coconut water
1 papaya

Estimated Totals:
Total Calories = 3,700
Total grams protein = 160g
Total grams of carbohydrates = 585g
Total grams of fats = 80g
Total water consumption = 112 ounces (factoring in water for
protein drinks too)

Robert's Recap on creating a Successful Nutrition Program

To be successful in your nutrition program, you will have to really clearly define what you want to accomplish and determine how hard you are willing to work to achieve it. You'll need to create a detailed vision, a timeline, and action plan, and then implement while consistently holding yourself account-able. You'll want to have a support network of those who believe in your aspirations almost as much as you believe in your ability to make your aspira-tions become realities. Athletic success goes hand-in-hand with a successful nutrition program and that has to be fully understood.

Whatever your vision, aspiration, or goal, commitment comes first. Some of us want to lose weight; some want to gain weight; some want to become successful bodybuilders; others want to tone up. Some of us want to become fitness models and make a career in the fitness industry; others of us want to change some bad habits so we can live longer and feel healthier. We each have a different approach, but the fundamental, foundational base of all of our aspirations is the same—a desire to achieve something. Achievement can be obtained by utilizing a program that is followed consistently through. When you determine what you want to do with your nutritional health, read back through some of the tips and suggestions based on those goals (be it mass-building, toning up, pre-contest dieting, or maintaining your current physique) and incorporate whatever material makes sense to you. Above all else, be-lieve in yourself sincerely and work hard for the changes you want to create in your life. You can do it because millions of people who didn't even think they could change their life have done exactly that. You already KNOW you can change your life and now you have a few extra tools, coupled with the inspiration and motivation you have within yourself to make it happen.

Document your transformation. It will be a lot of fun to show others later on and will be an inspirational tool to help others bring out the best in them-selves as well.

Robert's Top 10 tips to creating a Successful Nutrition Program

1. Have a really smart approach. If the food you are considering eating is known for its unhealthy reputation, it is probably something you'll want to avoid.

2. Ensure the majority of your diet is composed of nutrient-dense foods, such as plant-based "whole foods."

3. If it had a face, a family, and the ability to experience fear and pain, it isn't food. It is the remains of an animal that used to be alive and experience life just like we do. Eat the foods that caused the least amount of harm to be produced and "harvested" and you'll feel really good about your food choices everyday.

4. Drink sufficient amounts of water. The body is made up mostly of water, just like our muscles, so to maintain a healthy body and healthy muscles, consume a lot of water.

5. Focus on nourishment as your primary objective and choose the foods that provide the most nutrition for sustained energy, recovery from exercise, and for satiation and satisfaction so you don't over eat or under eat.

6. Keep your meal frequency fairly high. Eating often allows you to stay nourished all day long without feeling too hungry or too full and keeps your body burning fat quickly and your energy levels high.

7. Eat a variety of foods. It can be tough on a bodybuilding diet to include a lot of variety but make a strong effort to incorporate lots of different foods. It makes a bodybuilding diet so much more enjoyable.

8. Document your nutrition program. Keep a nutrition journal in addition to your training journal so you always have a record of what is working well, what isn't working well, and have it all on file to reference, evaluate, and reflect upon.

9. Be consistent in your nutrition program and keep yourself accountable. Most plateaus and stagnation periods in people's lives come from lack of accountability and lack of consistency. Make sure both of those aspects are considered and followed through. It's hard to improve if you're not putting in the work that leads to improvement. Consistency ensures forward progress, and accountability keeps you honest and makes you follow through.

10. Make a real, sincere, authentic, and honest effort to reach your nutrition goals. Most people just don't really try. Be one of the people that doesn't just say they want a change, but rather go out and create the change you want to experience.

"When I first found Robert and veganbodybuilding.com, I had previous weight training experience as a vegetarian. I knew how to structure my diet for optimal results. However, once I transitioned to veganism, I definitely needed help. Robert and the community at veganbodybuilding.com were very welcoming and supportive. I was able to ask questions, and I received valuable input. Without veganbodybuilding.com, I sincerely doubt that I would be making the progress that I am today.

Robert's attitude is amazing. No matter what life throws at him, he always exudes optimism and confidence. His upbeat attitude is contagious and very inspirational. He has put in tremendous effort to show the world that you can be vegan AND a successful bodybuilder. Thanks Robert for all of your hard work!"

Carrie Tanasichuk
VeganBodybuilding.com website member
Saskatchewan, Canada

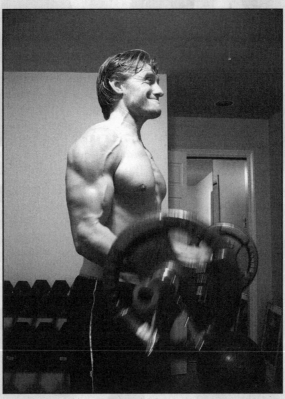

Training in Canada

Chapter 4

How to Create a Successful Training Program

"I love training more than anything else I do. You've got to if you want to be a bodybuilder. I love every exercise, you name it. Any exercise you give me, I take it as a challenge and I can make it my favorite. That's how you become a pro bodybuilder. You learn to love every rep of every exercise and treat it like its special."

Dennis James
IFBB Pro Bodybuilder

So now you want to be a bodybuilder. Where do you go from here? Creating a training program first starts with your own unique visions, goals, and ideas of what you expect to accomplish as a bodybuilder. Are you adopting this lifestyle to improve your health, to fulfill a lifelong dream, to build muscle, to change your physique for a role in a movie, to make money, to be a competitive athlete, to become a professional bodybuilder, or for some other reason? It matters not what your goal is but how you act on your goal and where you take it once you determine what you want to achieve.

Different goals will require different approaches and different training programs, but one thing that is universally understood is that lifting weights with intensity consistently results in muscle growth when properly supported with a solid nutrition and/or supplementation program. Simply putting in the time and intensity will yield results. Your specific results will depend on your objective, and the more clearly your objective is defined, the easier it will be to tailor your training program to your specific needs.

First of all, determine what your objective is. Once that has been established, start with a shell of basic exercises and movements that can become more intricate as your body adapts to the stress it is being put under. I always encourage people to start out easy with the basics. Like I wrote about in the Beginning Bodybuilding chapter, you're going to want to ease into a new program simply because it is additional physical stress that your body isn't used to, and you'll want to give your body the opportunity to adapt to the increased workload and respond in ways that fit your bodybuilding interests.

My real start to bodybuilding came from the Bill Phillips Body-For-LIFE program. That is the training program I was following on my own for a year before I met up with my friend Jordan who became my training partner. The Body-For-LIFE program was a specific type of training method I followed that had me training my upper body and lower body on alternating days and had me training with a certain level of intensity. The program included a lot of specifics regarding exercises and exercise styles such as incorporating super-sets. The program also required a level of accountability that ultimately led to success. Later on, I adopted a more traditional bodybuilding program that most bodybuilders follow, training one or two muscle groups per workout and only training that muscle group about once a week. That is the primary approach I have had over the past eight years and seems to be a bodybuilding program that I am comfortable with. Even within this approach I still have lots of different ways of training my body, including low repetitions, high reps, slow-speed reps, high intensity reps, short workouts, long workouts, partial reps, super-sets, drop-sets, etc. When I first followed the Body-For-LIFE program, my desire was just to get bigger. Now, my desire is to compete as a bodybuilder and that is how I train. Therefore, rather than follow a general fitness approach that works for "everybody," I follow my own bodybuilding program designed to work well for me. When I am consistent, it works well, and I continue to improve and achieve goals I set for myself. I always remain open to new ideas and new systems. Through working with personal trainers, I learn new approaches and apply them whenever they seem to make sense and fit into my current program.

Below is some information that I extracted from one of my other books *Your Personal Best*. This is a plan I created for some beginning bodybuilding programs and some additional strategies to support your bodybuilding lifestyle:

Pre-workout Fitness Basics

Warm-up

Before you begin exercising, it is always important to warm your body up. I do this in a variety of ways. When I exercise I wear athletic pants, a sweatshirt, and often a hat or knit cap to keep my body warm, even when I'm not moving. Even if it is in the middle of a hot summer in Oregon, I'm wearing my pants and sweatshirt in the gym to keep my muscles constantly warm. If I am driving to the gym, I turn the heat on the in the car to make my body warm up and even start sweating. Those are some ways that I warm-up before I actually physically exert myself. Traditional warm-up pre-workout exercises are jogging, running, sit-ups, push-ups, jumping jacks, or using some sort of cardiovascular equipment such as a treadmill, stationary bike, or a stair-stepper. Many gyms use obnoxious amounts of air conditioning, and that is the primary reason I wear warm clothing when I workout. If I'm training on Muscle Beach in Venice, CA during the spring or summertime, I won't wear a sweatshirt and pants. In fact, I enjoy wearing muscle shirts on Muscle Beach or no shirt at all. But since most fitness centers keep the inside temperature cool, I keep myself warm by the way I dress in the gym.

Regardless of whether you're preparing to lift weights, go for a bike ride, or play a game of soccer, it is always important to warm-up your body by doing low-intensity aerobic and anaerobic movements. I primarily lift weights, but I also engage in fun sports activities too. I play soccer and basketball on occasion and even dance. My warm-up preparation for all physical activity is fairly similar. My standard warm-up lasts about 5-10 minutes. Usually by then, I feel a lot of blood flowing through my body. My body feels warm; my muscles and joints are loose; flexibility has increased, and my lungs are actively engaged.

My personal pre-workout warm-up commonly consists of jogging, stair running, or stair climbing, sit-ups, push-ups, and jumping jacks or jumping rope (or replicating the jump rope movement without a rope). I like the running movements because it gets my whole body engaged, gets my lungs warmed up, and makes me start to sweat a bit. I like the stair running or climbing because it gets my lower body engaged in weight-bearing activity and helps warm up my lower body muscles. I do push-ups to warm up my upper-body muscles that are used in nearly every exercise, and I do sit-ups to get my core warmed up. Jumping jacks are incorporated at the end of my warm-up to start sweating. I only spend about two minutes on each pre-workout warm-up exercise. I have injured myself a number of times when I failed to warm-up before exercise, and I am sure you have experienced the same. Make it a point to warm up before you push yourself physically. Once you've warmed up, it's a good idea to do some light stretching as you ease into your workout.

Stretching

Contrary to popular belief, stretching should be done after warming up. Often times I see people stretching before jogging or doing anything to warm up the body. That approach can be dangerous for muscles, tendons, ligaments, and joints that are more easily stretched when they have been warmed up. I studied anatomy and physiology intensively and worked as a licensed massage therapist (LMT) for years so this is something I understand well. Blood needs to flow to areas of the body before the origin and insertion of a given muscle can be pulled or stretched. Otherwise it risks being damaged or injured. Be sure that you engage in warming up your body before you attempt to stretch any muscles, especially large muscles like hamstrings and quads which are involved in everyday movements and will hinder everything else you're doing if they get injured.

Once properly warmed up, stretch the muscles that you'll be primarily using in your workout as well as secondary muscles that may be called upon during the workout. Even when I'm training my legs, I still stretch my arms, back, and chest because leg workouts can mean total body workouts, and the whole body should be ready. Any time we're picking up a dumbbell or barbell or weight plate, we're using a whole variety of muscles, not just the muscle group we're training. It is a good idea to stretch out the whole body to reduce your risk of injury and to give yourself the best opportunity to succeed in your exercise program. Stretch during the workout as well to open up more blood flow and to lengthen the muscles providing a greater range of motion and better overall flow of movement.

Another excellent time to stretch is after the workout. This benefits athletes of all types and is something I personally resolve to focus more time on in the future. Post-workout stretching is great for the muscles and will often provide lasting results of looser, suppler muscles that are more flexible, have a greater range of motion, and are at a lesser risk for injury.

When you've warmed up, stretched out, and are ready to begin exercising, proceed to more challenging movements as the workout progresses.

General Fitness Basics (no special equipment required):

When it comes to general fitness, the basics are often the best and most effective exercises. There are plenty of high-tech machines and pieces of equipment out there, but nothing seems to match the benefits of running, jumping, swimming, cycling, climbing, pushing, and pulling in their simplest forms.

A lot can be accomplished without any special equipment at all. I've led fitness classes using no equipment whatsoever, performing exercises using bodyweight and have exhausted participants and myself as a result. We all have the capacity and ability to push ourselves physically just by doing basic exercises using our own body mechanics. Have you ever tried doing multiple sets of chin-ups or pull-ups, for example? Just doing five sets of pull-ups to exhaustion with each set will wipe out most people, and that is often just a warm-up for one of my workouts. The same can be said for bodyweight dips, or push-ups, bodyweight squats, lunges, static holds, and explosive jumps or sprints. Some of the most grueling workouts of my life involved no equipment whatsoever but involved running 400-meter sprints up steep hills, running repeated sets of 1000-meter sprints at maximum effort, sprinting up stadium stairs, explosive plyometric circuits, and bodyweight exercises like squats and lunges to failure.

The most exhausting workouts of my life were during cross country and track practice in high school and college which demanded every ounce of energy I had. Soccer conditioning camps and endurance races from my days as a runner were incredibly physically demanding and exhausting. Special gym club equipment is nice and is something I prefer as a bodybuilder who spends five days a week in a gym, but there are many effective exercises that can be completed literally anywhere.

Here is a list of some non-equipment exercises to incorporate into your exercise program. If you are not familiar with one or more of these exercises by name, search it on the Internet to get a description (and often photos and videos) of what they are.

Endurance and Lower Body Exercises:

Walking
Jogging
Running
Sprinting
Hiking
Jumping
Climbing
Squats
Lunges
Wall sits
Stair climbing
Box jumps
Jumping rope
Lateral side-steps

Upper Body Exercises

Chin-ups
Pull-ups
Dips
Push-ups
Static holds
Hand stands
Wall push-ups
Bridge push-ups
Lifting heavy objects
Bouldering and rock climbing
Pushing or pulling movements

Core Exercises

Crunches
Sit-ups
Leg lifts and leg raises
Bridge static holds
Yoga poses and movements
Pilates movements and exercises

Total Body Exercises

Yoga poses and movements
Jumping jacks
Star Jumps
Running
Sprinting
Mountain climbing
Sequence of a squat to a push-up to a jump, repeated
Cross-Fit exercises using body mechanics only

With all of those exercises, you can no longer use the excuse that you don't have a gym membership for a reason not to exercise. There are many more non-equipment exercises that you can do which aren't listed here, including any aerobics movements, yoga poses, Pilates movements, dance, martial arts, and traditional exercises that don't involve a gym but could be performed if you have access to a bike for cycling or a pool for swimming. In this case of non-equipment exercise, playing chess and playing poker don't count, even if they are on television's sports networks. Though extremely mentally stimulating, and I enjoy both, they won't aid in getting you into shape; but running up hills, doing lunges in your yard, sprints and pull-ups in the park, and sit-ups and push-ups on your living room floor will. Just put the activities into action and watch your body transform naturally.

Create a program using those exercises that will keep you exercising 3-5 days a week for 30-90 minutes at a time. Alter your program as you adapt and progress and incorporate other aspects into your training such as team sports and weight lifting.

General Weight Training Basics

When it comes to weight training, always begin by learning how the equipment works before you attempt to use it. Make sure that you know its proper function and what it is designed to do before you incorporate it into your program. The general idea is that any exercise should be a controlled movement without a lot of jerking of the body or allowing gravity or momentum to take over. A typical rule practiced by many is to decide on a muscle group or groups to train, pick out desired exercises, and begin by warming up and stretching before engaging in the exercises. Once the first exercise is determined, it is common to do at least one warm-up set if not more, using high repetitions to get the muscles, joints, ligaments, and tendons familiar with the stress they will be under for the ensuing 60 minutes at the gym. I like to begin with a very controlled movement to start my workout. Let's say I'm training my arms, for example. If I am about to start training my biceps, I'll usually pick some light dumbbells and do two sets of 15-30 repetitions of bicep curls before I begin my actual workout. When it comes to my working sets, I will do 8-12 repetitions. The general rule is to warm up with a couple of sets on low weight and high reps before pushing it hard. I've been known to do as many as 50-100 reps for some muscle groups with very light weight simply as a warm-up for that muscle group, which in my mind is equivalent to running before a leg exercise.

A fairly common standard is to do 15-30 sets per workout. That is quite a large scale, but it depends on the person, the muscles being trained, the experience level, the goals, etc. What I do is pick out about five different exercises for a given workout and do 3-5 sets per exercise which equals 15-25 overall sets. Let's say for this example, I'm training my chest for the day. The entire workout may look like this:

Warm-up

Stretch

Two sets of 25 push-ups and two sets of dumbbell chest press as additional warm-up targeting the muscles I'll be training.

Dumbbell Chest Press x 4 sets

Incline Dumbbell Flys x 4 sets

Decline Barbell Bench Press x 4 sets

Dips x 4 sets

Cable crossovers x 3 sets

Total = 19 sets

For each of those sets, I aim for the standard 8-12 repetitions. Depending on my specific focus, I may do as few as 3-5 reps or as many as 15-20 reps, but I often target that optimal muscle-building range between 8-12 reps per set.

With my personal workouts I usually spend 45-90 seconds rest between sets for small muscle groups like biceps, triceps, chest, shoulders, and back. I rest 120-180 seconds between sets when I train larger muscles such as my quads, hamstrings, and glutes—powerful lower body muscles that require longer rest periods to recover from the exercise. Sometimes I even spend up to five minutes rest if I am doing 900-pound leg presses, for example. Chest and back could be considered somewhere in the middle, being larger than arms and smaller than legs, and depending on the exercises, especially heavy chest press or heavy bent-over rows, I do spend closer to 120-180 seconds of rest for those larger upper body muscles, if not a full five minutes when trying to reach a 1-rep max personal best lift on say flat bench press.

There are variations in range of motion from full range of motion to partial range of motion. They all have their own purposes and functions, but I prefer as often as possible to do full range of motion to try to get the most out of the exercise. Using a spotter, someone to watch you and assist you in moving the weight if need be when using free weights, is recommended. Having a spotter or training partner takes away some of the worry of injury or worry of getting stuck in the middle of the movement and allows you to focus more on completing the reps and getting benefit from the exercise. In addition to general training sets and reps, there are also super-sets, drop-sets, burn-out sets, and partial reps that can be performed. I will briefly explain each of them as I understand them.

Super-Sets – Super-sets can be described as completing a different exercise for the same muscle group immediately after the completion of the primary exercise. An example would be training chest doing bench press to failure and immediately, without rest, doing incline dumbbell press. The idea is to engage any muscle fibers that may have been missed in the primary exercise and to burn out that muscle group. It feels really good too. A common super-set for chest is push-ups. As soon as you finish a set of dips, chest press, or any other chest exercise, immediately drop to the floor and do some push-ups. This can be done for any muscle group. Note that your muscles will be very fatigued, so choose an exercise that you won't need a spotter for, one that you can set the weight down anytime your muscles give out and still be safe. For example, you wouldn't want to do squats as your super-set exercise. The risk of muscles giving out and the risk of injury are too high. Squats would likely be your primary exercise, and leg curls or leg extensions would be your super-set exercise. With chest, you wouldn't want a free-weight bench press as your super-set exercise, but a machine bench-press would be optimal. If you have a spotter, the free-weight bench press would be okay, but something as powerful as squats should be avoided as a super-set exercise even if a spotter is present. In almost all cases of super-sets, you will be doing a less strenuous exercise than the primary exercise, and you will be using less weight for your super-set exercise than you normally would because you will already be fatigued from the primary exercise. If you normally use 30-pound dumbbells for bicep curls but are doing dumbbell bicep curls as a super-set after barbell bicep curls, you'll probably want use 20-pound dumbbells or even 15-pound dumbbells since you'll already be fatigued from the primary exercise you completed to failure immediately before.

Drop-Sets – Drop-sets are when you complete an exercise, strip off some weight, and immediately do the same exercise. You follow that routine for a few sets. It is very common and also a fun style of training. A common example is training biceps doing straight bar bicep curls. When you complete your set with 80 pounds, you immediately drop to 60 pounds; do as many reps as possible, then drop to 40 pounds; do as many reps as possible and drop to 20 pounds. Finish doing as many reps as you can. Your muscles will be burning, you'll have funny expressions on your face, but you'll enjoy it. You may feel silly gritting your teeth and grimacing with a 20-pound bar, but you will know that you have pushed it very hard. It's perfectly normal and expected that you'll look like a wimp when really you're not. Drop-sets are designed to trigger all muscle fibers big and small and to burn out the muscle, stimulating growth.

My very favorite are leg press drop-sets. I perform these with the help of my trainer at the gym, Cesar Martinez. We put six or seven 45-pound plates on either side of the leg press sled, and I do a set to failure. He takes one plate off at a time, and I perform the next set with only about five seconds of rest in between. He doesn't take one plate off of each side between sets but literally just one plate. It is the most grueling experience I have had in the gym because we're talking 14 consecutive drop-sets to empty the leg press sled. Halfway through, my glutes become numb, and sometimes I'll even whimper or want to cry, but I make it through. I can't always finish the entire set and occasionally have to stop before the full set is complete because the intensity, burn, and pain is too much to handle. When I leave the gym on those days, I feel extra proud of the mental strength it took to get through that type of workout. Sometimes I even vomit, but that is what true intensity can lead to. I think it makes Cesar proud of how hard he is pushing me and how much he is challenging me. I suggest incorporating drop-sets yourself on occasion and experience the addiction to pain that may ensue.

Burn-out Sets – Burn-out sets are simply workout sets where you do as many reps as possible until you can't do anymore. They can be for any exercise and any muscle group. You can do a burn-out set of lunges until you literally fall over, or a burn-out set of push-ups until you fall flat on your face, or any other exercise you desire. Again, it is important to choose an exercise that can be controlled and that you can stop at anytime, much like super-sets. Don't do a burn-out set of bench press without a spotter or you will end up with the barbell and weight lying across your chest. Burn-out sets are designed to do what the name insinuates, burn-out the muscle. These are usually done at the very end of a workout, primarily for the psychological benefit of leaving everything you have in the gym, making it feel like your entire workout was a burn-out. It has a physical benefit too—exhausting all your muscles, ensuring a productive workout, and guaranteeing progress.

Partial Reps – Partial reps are reps that are not completed to the full range of motion. They allow you to use more weight than if you had to do the full range of motion. It results in you being stronger, as you're able to manage more weight. Common exercises for partial reps are partial squats, partial dead-lifts, partial shoulder press, partial bench press, partial arm or leg curls, and rack pulls, which are partial rows similar to shrugs. They help you build up strength and help you put on muscle size. I don't do a lot of partial reps with the exception of the end of a set when I am too fatigued to complete the full rep. I keep the set going by doing a few partial reps, fully burning out my muscles. Many power lifters use partial reps and partial movements to practice explosive exercises or to get more familiar with a specific aspect of the exercise. Sometimes partial reps are simply used to improve grip strength.

Explore your gym to get familiar with the equipment and start a basic weight-training program. Use basic movements, free weights, and machines. Seek out the assistance of a personal trainer if you wish to further enhance your weight lifting experience. I give my personal trainer Cesar a lot of credit for the development of my physique because even though I've been training for a decade, I learn something new each and every time we train together. He also helps push me harder, challenges me to not give up when pain and fatigue start to set in, and helps me bring out the best in my physique. He gives me advice, gives me feedback, keeps me accountable, and is fun to work with. My friend Ed Bauer, who is also a vegan bodybuilder, is a personal trainer at the same gym as Cesar in Portland, OR. Ed and I often train together and push each other to new record lifts. Look up Cesar Martinez or Ed Bauer if you're in the Portland area. They will push you hard and help you achieve your fitness goals. They have helped me big time!

A basic weight-training program will help you get stronger, more fit, and more toned. Weight training often puts you in a good mood, creates motivation and inspiration in other aspects of your life, and can be a great social or group activity. For more information on the subject of creating exercise programs, seek out books, magazines, websites, and articles dedicated to weight training and have fun getting in awesome shape! Please join our online forum community on www.veganbodybuilding.com as well. I've met most of my best friends and current training partners on that website forum.

Bodybuilding Basics:

To be a successful bodybuilder, you need to first start with the basics and be patient and allow your progress to take place. You must understand that results do not come overnight. To achieve a desired look you have to put in the time and dedication and commit yourself to hard work.

Bodybuilding basics include creating a workout schedule and sticking to it. This doesn't mean doing the same exercises; it means training consistently with purpose and having a specific vision in mind. It means going to the gym even on the days you don't really feel like it. It means making time to stay on schedule and stay on track. Don't ever say, "I ran out of time to train today." Make time. We all have 1,440 minutes in a day. What are you doing with your time? Plan ahead; sleep an hour less; pack meals with you; wake up early and go to the gym before work; stop watching TV, and stop surfing the Internet. Make every moment count. Work hard to make time for fitness because the results are worth it.

The basics of bodybuilding also include an understanding of the role that a sound nutritional program plays in the progression of your physique trans- formation. Nutrition is a key element in bodybuilding, perhaps the most important and most overlooked component in the whole bodybuilding lifestyle. Other basics to remember are the exercises themselves. There are a few somewhat primitive power exercises that do more for you than any of the new-age equipment that is floating around late night television infomercials or at your hipster health club. These basic exercises will be the foundation of your training and include squats, bench press, dead lifts, clean and jerk, over- head press, leg press, chin-ups, barbell bicep curls, lunges, hanging leg raises, bent-over rows, dips, dumbbell curls, lateral raises, and shrugs. You don't need cables or complicated machines for these exercises; you just need the basic equipment and a sense of determination and you will succeed in body- building.

Efficiency is another important component to the basics of bodybuilding. This means that you don't have to spend two or three hours in the gym to get desired results, but you can achieve the same results by training smarter and more efficiently, staying focused while you're at the gym. This doesn't mean that you have to stuff yourself full of food at each meal until you can't possi- bly eat anymore. Efficiency means understanding what actions need to take place to enable your body and your body's systems to perform on optimum levels. Train just as much as you need to, not more. If you spend too much time in the gym, you will break down muscle fibers at a faster rate than they are recovering, and this could lead to over training or injury. Spend about an hour to 90 minutes of weight training during your session. Any more con- secutive time spent weight training can be counter-productive. You can get away with 90-minute workouts for some larger muscle groups, but in most cases that full amount of time in a single weight training session is not neces- sary. Allow yourself 45-180 seconds rest between sets, depending on the muscles being trained, noting the larger muscles will need more rest between sets. Sticking to this plan, you should be fresh to continue your workout full of energy. Being efficient will keep you ahead of the game, and assist in your overall bodybuilding progress.

Supplementation can be a major factor in bodybuilding. Again, there are countless options out there for products that could possibly enhance your physique, but stick to the basics and you will reap plenty of benefits. Protein is one of the most popular supplements you can take. Take a protein shake in the morning and another one after your workout or at night time, and you should accumulate all the protein you need, assuming you are eating plenty of foods throughout the day. You can take many more protein drinks, as is suggested in some of the meal programs, but it isn't necessary. Taking a multivitamin is another common practice and a great idea for everyone, not just bodybuilders. Multivitamins help bring up levels of certain nutrients you may be lacking in your diet from day to day. Liquid forms tend to be the most effective because they are absorbed the fastest and are the most bio-available. This means your body uses a higher percentage of the nutrients than it does from other forms such as pills or powders. Amino acid L-glutamine is another very popular supplement for bodybuilders. L-glutamine is the most important amino acid in muscle recovery and growth and becomes "essential" for bodybuilders trying to make the most gains with the help of effective supplementation. There are plenty of basic supplements such as Vitamin C and anti-oxidants to promote a strong immune system and omega 3 and 6 essential fatty acids from hemp, flax, or other preferred plant-based sources. Branched-chain amino acids, creatine, nitric oxide, meal replacement powders, and other popular bodybuilding supplements can be used as well. Research your options, but stick to the basics as often as possible. Supplements can be a nutritional short cut of sorts, but don't sacrifice quality in place of quick results. Look for the highest quality, most natural supplements out there and choose the ones that make the most logical sense to you and then apply them as you wish into your bodybuilding program. Visit www.veganproteins.com for a variety of vegan supplements.

Setting specific goals and visions is not only a crucial component to a bodybuilding program but is also another bodybuilding basic. You don't train without motivation, do you? There has to be something that drives you to push your body hard or push it to its physical limit. For many bodybuilders, the thought of a chiseled, fit, strong, aesthetically pleasing physique is enough to make them train without fear of pain or failure. Whatever your reasons are, make your visions clear and as specific as possible. Tell others about the things you desire, and show them the work ethic that it takes to achieve greatness in a demanding sport. You can make a career out of bodybuilding by being a marketable representative and ambassador to products, companies, brands, and organizations. That is one of the ways bodybuilding benefited me on a personal and professional level. It can be yours to experience if you write it into your vision and work hard to achieve it.

Following the basics of bodybuilding will not only enhance your physique but also your overall bodybuilding program. You will become more efficient in your workouts and more effective in your nutrition programs. Stick to the basics and you will become extraordinary.

If weight training is on your list of interests, below is a sample weight-training program I took from my own training schedule. The numbers represent the sets and reps (Example 1x10 would be 1 set for 10 reps).

1 Week Sample Weight Training Program

Day 1 - Chest and Biceps

Chest

Flat bench dumbbell press 1x12, 1x10, 1x8

Decline barbell bench press 1x12, 1x10, 1x8

Incline barbell bench press 1x12, 1x10, 1x8

Cable crossovers 1x12, 1x10, 1x8

Biceps

Barbell bicep curls 1x12, 1x10, 1x8

Alternating dumbbell hammer curls 1x12, 1x10, 1x8

Dumbbell concentration curls 1x12, 1x10, 1x8

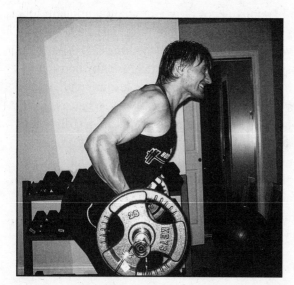

Training in Canada

Day 2 Back and Abs

Back

Chin-ups 1x12, 1x10, 1x8
T-bar rows 1x12, 1x10, 1x8
Dead lifts 1x12, 1x10, 1x8
Cable rows 1x12, 1x10, 1x8

Abs

Hanging leg raises 1x20, 1x20, 1x20
Cable pull-downs 1x20, 1x20, 1x20
Front and side crunches 1x20, 1x20, 1x20

Day 3 REST

Day 4 Shoulders and Triceps

Shoulders

Dumbbell lateral raises 1x12, 1x10, 1x8
Seated military press 1x12, 1x10, 1x8
Over-head dumbbell shoulder press 1x12, 1x10, 1x8
Front cable or dumbbell raises 1x12, 1x10, 1x8

Triceps

Rope triceps pull-downs 1x12, 1x10, 1x8
Skull crushers (French press) 1x12, 1x10, 1x8
Dumbbell kickbacks 1x12, 1x10, 1x8
Dips 1x12, 1x10, 1x8

Day 5 LEGS

Leg extensions 1x12, 1x10, 1x8
Squats 1x12, 1x10, 1x8, 1x6
Leg press 1x12, 1x10, 1x8
Hack squat 1x12, 1x10, 1x8
Lying hamstring curl 1x12, 1x10, 1x8
Standing calf raises 1x20, 1x15, 1x12

Day 6 REST

* Cardiovascular training if desired.

Day 7 REST

1 week sample training program <u>without weights</u> or exercise equipment

Day 1

Run for 3 miles at a moderate pace

Push-ups 1x20, 1x20, 1x20, 1x20, 1xfailure

Sit-ups 1x30, 1x30, 1x30, 1x 30, 1xfailure

Yoga poses or static holds for upper body for 10 minutes, with rest between sets

General stretching

Day 2

Stair running for 20 minutes

Lunges 1x30, 1x30, 1x30, 1xfailure

Bodyweight squats 1x20, 1x25, 1x30, 1xfailure

Star jumps 1x20, 1x20, 1x20

Wall-sits for 10 minutes, rest between sets

Day 3 REST

Day 4

Walk briskly for 40 minutes

Decline push-ups (feet up on a bench) 1x20, 1x20, 1x20, 1xfailure

Narrow hand position push-ups 1x20, 1x20, 1x20, 1xfailure

Chin-ups 1xfailure, 1xfailure, 1xfailure, 1xfailure

Dips 1xfailure, 1xfailure, 1xfailure, 1xfailure

General stretching

Day 5

Run for 5 miles at a moderate pace

40-meter sprints x 5

100-meter up-hill sprints x 3

Jumping jacks or jumping rope 1x20, 1x30, 1x40, 1x50

General stretching

Day 6

Cycling for 45 minutes

Yoga poses and stretching

Day 7 REST

To see demonstrations of those exercises listed in either the weight training sample program or the non-weight sample program or to learn what they are if you are not familiar with them, you can do basic searches on the Internet to get all of your questions answered.

Post-exercise suggestions and recommendations to better health and fitness

In addition to exercise itself, there are other great ways of supporting your fitness lifestyle that are recommended. Incorporating some of these modalities can help improve your overall level of health.

Massage Therapy

As someone who worked as a licensed massage therapist for years specializing in sports massage therapy, I recommend getting a massage on a fairly regular basis to greatly benefit you in a variety of ways. Massage therapy helps increase circulation throughout the body, helps soften tense and tight muscles, helps prevent injury, and helps with greater range of motion and flexibility. Getting a deep-tissue or sports massage every month, if not more frequently, is a great way to keep your body in top form so it can perform at a high level while you exercise and compete. It will also allow you to reduce stress, focus on breathing and relaxation, improve posture, reduce chronic pain, and even improve muscle tone. I have had the opportunity throughout my career as a massage therapist to work with the US Olympic Speed Skating Team, with professional athletes, and with avid weekend warriors who were relieved from their chronic pain after working with me. I've seen and experienced first-hand the great work that massage therapy can do for athletes and non-athletes alike. I currently get bodywork from Jen Fichter, LMT in Portland, OR who is an outstanding therapist and a friend for whom I have a lot of admiration and respect.

Hydrotherapy, Cryotherapy, and Alternating Temperature Therapies

The use of heat and ice after exercise, before exercise, or during off days from exercise is another healthy way to keep your body functioning well. Heat from saunas, steam rooms, or hot tubs helps muscles loosen and stay soft; it allows the body to sweat, increases circulation, and brings blood to an area that is directly in contact with the heat which allows greater flexibility and greater range of motion. An excellent time to stretch muscles is while in a sauna or steam room. Cryotherapy, the use of ice, is a great way to reduce inflammation to an area of the body that has had some sort of trauma. Cryotherapy treats swelling and cools sore, inflamed muscles. Using heat and ice treatments in conjunction with massage therapy is an excellent way to keep your body healthy, strong, and injury free. I use hydrotherapy, cryotherapy, and alternating heat therapies on a regular basis. I enjoy steam rooms and saunas the most and find it beneficial to my overall health and wellness. I also relied heavily on ice for hours a day when I had major lower back soreness, and it helped out dramatically.

Chiropractic Adjustments

Physical activity may cause the body to fall out of alignment. Chiropractic work can adjust it back to normal. Chiropractic work helped me through some specific circumstances in 2001, 2008, and 2009. I received some chiropractic adjustments from Dr. Ron Six in Phoenix, AZ in 2001 when I injured my back doing squats while training for a bodybuilding competition. I was in Hawaii in November 2008 competing at the Raw Games (www.rawgames.org), and I threw my back out in such a way that I could barely walk or sit. While in Hawaii, some of the coordinators at the Raw Games spotted my injury and drove me up to one of the resort cabins, and a massage therapist worked on my muscles for ten to fifteen minutes. Chiropractic Doctor John Peck, who was heading up the surfing competition at the Raw Games, manipulated my spine, explaining his actions every step of the way. He informed me that two of my lower lumbar vertebrae had been rotated causing nerve tendon damage which was leading to all of my pain and limited range of motion. Dr. Peck voluntarily worked with me for about an hour, adjusting my entire spine and informing me of what he was doing through the entire process to ease my worries and to create a comforting environment. When he completed his work, I slowly sat up, and then stood up and walked around feeling incredible. Just an hour earlier I could barely bend over to sit and was in a great deal of pain. Hours later I was dancing out on the grass jamming with musicians Cipes and the People and Singing Bear. Normally it takes weeks or months to get comfortable again with exercise, especially lifting weights when I injure my back in that way, but I was back in action immediately, and I appreciate the work that Dr. Peck volunteered to help me recover.

I have a whole new respect for Chiropractic work and will be incorporating it into my current bodybuilding competition preparation more often in the future. Just recently, in the spring of 2009, I again injured my back. I was unable to walk, and it was in fact more severe than my injury in Hawaii that left me barely able to walk. Just climbing in and out of the front seat of my car took minutes and walking from my car to my front door (about 20 feet), was not possible without a rest in between. I worked with multiple Portland-based chiropractors including Dr. Jason Lindekugel. I went from not being able to walk to getting up on the bodybuilding stage eight days later and becoming the 2009 INBA Northwestern USA Natural Bodybuilding Champion. It was an incredible feeling. I still have some lower back issues stemming back from my teenage years of athletic injuries and from painful weight lifting accident injuries in 2001 and 2003, but with the help of some chiropractic doctors, I have been able to overcome the pain and injuries and have experienced athletic success and achievement.

Give chiropractors a try; they could really take a load off your back.

Yoga – Pilates - Meditation

Though there are books with great lengths that talk about these topics individually, I'm grouping them together because I don't know a whole lot about them individually. However, I have experienced all of them and know that they are great additions to any fitness program. These forms of relaxation, training, stretching, and focus help the mind and body get to a relaxed place and a place of better health through the movements involved in their practice. If you haven't tried any of them or the many other forms of alternative exercise and post-exercise conditioning, I suggest you give each a try and find out which one resonates the best with you and incorporate it into your lifestyle on occasion. It's a great way to add more variety and balance to your wellness program. One of my best friends who inspired me to be a successful writer, Ravi Raman, is a Yoga teacher, and you can read about his experiences on www.sethigherstandards.com. You will also be highly motivated because he is a motivational teacher and a seasoned personal development student. If you're already an athlete, it's no big stretch to give yoga a try.

Now that you are armed with a plethora of fitness suggestions, it is time to put your arms into action. Experiment with a variety of programs and find comfort in the ones that suit you best. Have fun feeling well and being fit!

Feel free to use my website www.veganbodybuilding.com as a resource for bodybuilding and fitness, plant-based nutrition, and motivation and inspiration as you begin or continue on your journey to improved health.

Robert's Recap for Creating a Successful Training Program

Creating a successful training program is just as important as creating a successful nutrition program. When you have both of them implemented and working in your favor, you are bound to be successful. Success usually breeds enjoyment, which enhances quality of life. You can see how important a solid training program can be. It can change your life in amazing ways. Learn a lot about the human body and know the importance of taking care of it through proper warm-ups and training methods, through sufficient nutrition and supplement intake, and through adequate rest and a positive attitude. You'll find that a sincere belief in yourself and an attitude that supports your aspirations could be something that makes a huge impact on your levels of success. Discover what your goals are and come up with an approach to support your ambitions and consistently follow through in deliberate actions that yield results. Enjoy the journey because if it isn't fun, it becomes a chore. As with everything else, keep a detailed journal of your progress. It will be something fun to look back on years down the road when you reminisce about the humble beginnings of your early bodybuilding days.

Robert's Top 10 tips to Creating a Successful Training Program

1. Act like a bodybuilder. Don't expect bodybuilding results if you're not willing to work like a bodybuilder to achieve them.

2. Always have a plan in mind and make sure your efforts everyday are in line with your plan for success.

3. Find meaning and passion in your training and in your bodybuilding lifestyle so you will look forward to it everyday. Otherwise, it will be something you dread or fear.

4. Keep yourself inspired by any means necessary. Find a training part-
    ner, hire a personal trainer, take progress photos, do whatever it takes
    to keep you inspired to improve. It is through improvement that one
    often finds fulfillment.

5. Learn from others who have been successful bodybuilders. There is
    no better way to learn about bodybuilding than by others who have
    done it and by doing it yourself.

6. Make bodybuilding a priority in your life. It doesn't have to be your
    #1 priority. If you're married, for example, it had better not be your
    #1 priority or you may not be married very long. Make the body-
    building lifestyle fairly high on your list of things that are important in
    your life and you will respect it, appreciate it, and be successful at it.

7. Set some really specific bodybuilding goals so you have detailed des-
    tinations to work toward—be it a competition, a certain amount of
    weight lifted, or a consecutive scheduled workout streak that you aim
    for; the more specific and detailed the goals, the better focus you'll
    have and harder you'll work to achieve them.

8. Create a timeline for success rather than a deadline. Deadlines are
    "all or nothing" while timelines can be adjusted based on progress.
    Timelines are much more effective in my experience, and I suggest
    you use them in your approach to bodybuilding.

9. Get a pen and paper and list your favorite aspects of the bodybuilding
    lifestyle. Only list your very favorite things that are very positive and
    get you excited about bodybuilding and weight training. Post the list
    somewhere you can see it daily as a reminder of why you do what
    you do. In this sport that is so tough mentally, physically, and psy-
    chologically, sometimes we need reminders of why we keep going
    when times get really challenging.

10. Have fun and share your bodybuilding success with others. This
    could likely inspire others around you. You may even get a new train-
    ing partner out of it because often you'll motivate people to come
    along and train with you to learn how to experience some of the same
    fulfillment and success you do on a daily basis.

"Before I came across Robert's website, I assumed that I was pretty much alone in terms of being a vegan who lifted weights. That seems crazy now looking back, because even I had been affected by that stereotype to the point that I believed it was unusual for some reason, a stereotype that I now think of as utterly foolish.

Robert has gone out of his way to promote the lifestyle and to gather other vegans together by becoming a positive role model. I've been impressed by his attitude and hard work over the years. He's constantly working, often too hard. Prior to knowing him, I had used non-vegan bodybuilding sources of information and veganized them to suit myself, but it has made things easier with a community of people who are already vegan. And it's especially good to follow Robert's progress and, due to his dedication, he is able to inspire in terms of what he has achieved in bodybuilding and also in mental attitude and determination."

Richard Watts
VeganBodybuilding.com Administrator,
Website/Graphic Designer - godfist.com/chrysander.com
United Kingdom

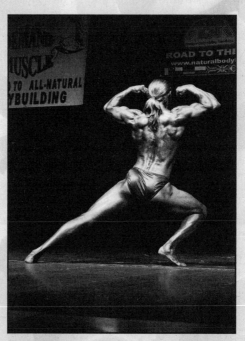

Robert winning the 2009 INBA Northwestern
USA Natural Bodybuilding Championships
(photo by Randall Perez – RandallPerez.com)

Chapter 5

The Most Important Lessons to be Learned and Followed in Bodybuilding

"The most important lesson I've learned is that the most productive exercises are simple and compound."

Markus Ruhl
IFBB Pro Bodybuilder

There are a few lessons I have learned about bodybuilding over the past ten years that are profoundly more important that others, and I feel it is important to outline some of those lessons. My intention is to save you a lot of time, save you from frustration, and teach you from my trials and errors in the bodybuilding industry.

1. Keep a journal to track your progress.

2. Be consistent. Consistency is key and is likely the biggest "make it or break it component."

3. Don't be so humble that you sell yourself short (think of the bigger picture).

4. Compete on stage; it's the best way to learn.

5. Work harder than anyone else you know.

1. Keep a journal to track your progress

Keep a journal to know what you're really doing in the gym and what you're not doing. Make it complete with a list of goals, progress notes, and workout details. Do the same for your nutrition program, keeping record of what you're eating, when, and in what quantities.

Training journals can be created and updated however you like. They can be very structured and have lists of all exercises performed, all food consumed, notes about how you were feeling, the supplements you took, what the weather was like, the time of day you exercised, etc. It all depends how detailed you want to be. I personally don't keep a meticulous journal, but I am a fan of keeping a journal in general and keeping track of progress to go back and reflect upon months or years later. It is such an effective tool for tracking and evaluating your progress or lack of progress and reveals a lot about you in ways you probably don't even anticipate.

I have been keeping an online journal on my www.veganbodybuilding.com website for the past three years. I update it with lists of goals, exercises, photos, and sometimes just text in short paragraph form sharing my thoughts for the day, my highs and lows, and my success and failures. I list the exercises I performed, the weight I used, the number of reps I completed, and other comments I share publicly in an online journal. To show how important and how significant keeping a journal can be, you can view the content from my three-year journal which is 70 pages long on this link: http://www.veganbodybuilding.com/phpBB2/viewtopic.php?f=24&t=2765 to see how much it means to me and my training progress.

It is really interesting and rewarding to go back down memory lane and review a training journal that I have kept online publicly for years. It has been viewed over 50,000 times on my website and has kept me going through the years of ups and downs as a competitive bodybuilder.

I have kept lots of different training journals over the years, some inspired by the Body-For-LIFE program and others I created on my own for my own personal records. The online journal on my website is very basic, but it does reveal a lot of my exercises, my emotions, and tells a story of some of the things I was doing throughout other areas of my life too. I find it to be worthwhile as I reflect back on it, but I also see the need for a more detailed format, something I will outline in this book.

I encourage everyone to keep a journal, whether public or private. Doing so can benefit many areas of your life, and I think it is worth the time invested each and every time a journal entry is made.

The key things to consider when keeping a journal are the following:

1. Record the date and even the time of day.

2. Record the exercises you completed along with the weights, reps, sets performed, and rest periods.

3.   Record the foods and supplements you consumed.

4. Include some notes about how you are feeling in general, what your goals were and what you achieved.

5. Make your journal consistent and update it frequently and accurately.

From my journal entries on my website you'll see that I may not have followed every single step with every journal entry, but that is a clear reason why my journal isn't as good as it could have been and displays some weaknesses that I can improve to make it even more effective. It also reflects the hectic and busy on-the-go lifestyle I lead which is supported by a lot of the text in my journal revealing the intensity of my "every moment counts" life. Given more time, or as I create more time, my journal may look a lot more like the following.

An example of an ideal journal looks like this:

Date: May 8, 2009   Time: 5:55PM

Today's Goals: State the goal of the day for your exercise program

Today's workout: Recap the actual workout that you performed

Warm-up:

Exercise   Minutes

Workout:

Exercise   Weight   Reps   Sets   Rest Period

Supplements:

Post-workout meals:

Notes/Comments:

The training journal can be made up in a spreadsheet or a word processing file that you can print out. On the following page is an example of a training log that you can photocopy and print out and use for yourself.

TRAINING JOURNAL

Date: _____   Time: _____

Today's Goals for the Workout: _____

_____

_____

Today's Summary of the Actual Workout: _____

_____

_____

Warm-up:

Exercise: _____   **Time:** _____

Workout:

Exercise	Weight	Sets	Reps	Rest Period

TRAINING JOURNAL

Supplements:

_____

_____

_____

_____

_____

Post-Workout Meals:

_____

_____

_____

_____

_____

Notes/Comments:

_____

_____

_____

_____

_____

_____

_____

The same style of journal can be used specifically for your nutrition program. I learned this from my early days following the Body-For-LIFE Program and used nutrition journals just as often as training journals.

NUTRITION JOURNAL

Date: _____

Today's Goals for the Nutrition Program:

_____

_____

Meal #	Time	Foods	Fluids	Approx Totals Calories	Protein	Fluid Oz.
1						
2						
3						
4						
5						
6						
7						
8						
Estimated Daily Totals:						

NUTRITION JOURNAL

Notes/Comments of Actual Nutrition Program:

_____

_____

_____

_____

_____

_____

_____

_____

_____

_____

_____

_____

_____

_____

_____

_____

_____

_____

_____

2. Be consistent. Consistency is key and is likely the biggest "make it or break it" component.

I know I write about consistency a lot, but it is for good reason. I really believe that consistency is the biggest key to success. Aside from having a clear vision to begin with, nothing is as important as consistency when it comes to achievement of anything, and I dedicate complete chapters to it in my other books and dedicate large segments of my motivational talks to this very subject.

Without consistency, there is no adaptation, there is no improvement, and there is no success. All it takes is some sort of accountability and application of consistent effort on a regular basis and success can be initiated and achieved. This is clearly evident in the sport of bodybuilding. The aspect of bodybuilding that nearly kept me out of the sport when I first started was precisely consistency. I had all the enthusiasm in the world, but I never even gave myself a fighting chance because I wasn't in the gym consistently enough to create any kind of change. I also wasn't eating consistently enough to support my bodybuilding ambitions.

If there is only one thing you learn from this chapter for success in the sport of bodybuilding (but also for success in life), it is to be consistent. Keeping training and nutrition journals supports consistency; having passion supports it; improving supports it directly; and making consistency second nature and implementing it supports it too. If you don't put in the time regularly, you won't improve, resulting only in frustration. But if you do put in the time, effort, intensity, and passion, and you do so regularly, you will improve, you will succeed, you will achieve, and you will be driven to keep that pattern going because of all the fun you are having and because of all the gains you are making. There is no better way to achieve this than through consistency. Keep yourself accountable and consistent, and give yourself a fighting chance to improve and succeed.

Some tips to keep yourself consistent in bodybuilding are the following:

1. Create a pattern to follow so you always know that you'll be able to fit your workouts in to your busy schedule. Train every day before work or after work or at a set time each day so you make it a priority. Find what works for you, but create a pattern to keep on schedule.

2. Workout with a training partner or a personal trainer so you have someone else counting on you to show up at the gym regularly.

3. Have a clear vision of what you plan to accomplish, and visualize your future success knowing that it is dependent on the time you spend in the gym and the effort that you put into bodybuilding.

4. Tell people about your intentions or make them public on a website. If you write down or verbally tell someone that you are going to the gym, it will help you stick with it because you'll feel guilty if you don't go. This reaffirms your commitment and will help you get to the gym even on days you don't really feel like it.

5. Use supplements to support your bodybuilding program so you can take a few shortcuts to success. Take in protein powders, essential fats, vitamins, minerals, and muscle-enhancing supplements that are vegan and natural. Watch your progress speed up and watch your motivation increase as a result.

6. Share your success with others and explain how you came to your achievements. Those explanations and conversations will reinforce in your own mind what it took to get there, and you'll naturally want to be just as consistent to keep the success going.

7. Make friends at the gym either with employees or members or both. When you have a community of people grow accustomed to seeing you, they will expect to see you often and regularly and will likely comment about your absence if you're away too long. This can help fuel motivation without feeling an intense obligation or having too much expectation on your shoulders. It can serve as a friendly reminder to drop in to train to see your friends.

8. Make bodybuilding fun. Not just working out, but eating, supplementing, posing, and everything that is involved in the bodybuilding lifestyle. Life is supposed to be enjoyable, and if bodybuilding is a 24-hour per day sport, it had better be fun or it simply isn't worth it. If you can find meaning in what you're doing and find fun in the bodybuilding lifestyle, you'll want to be more consistent to support your life's passion.

9. Join a community of athletes either in your city or online. Being part of a community that shares ideas and supports its members is a sure way to keep you going and bring more excitement to your bodybuilding life.

10. Take 'before" photos and continue to take "progress" photos every couple of months as you embark on a bodybuilding program or as you continue to progress as a long-time bodybuilder. "Before" and "after" photos are great motivators to keep you consistent, provided you are making inspirational progress.

3. Don't be so humble that you sell yourself short (think of the bigger picture).

The general public may often view bodybuilders as cocky, arrogant, or self-absorbed. Perhaps that is a bit of an assumption on my part, but I've been around the industry long enough to know there is some sort of truth in that common generalization of bodybuilders as seen by the mainstream public. The counter reaction of a bodybuilder is to be humble, to go against the stereotype that they fear they will fall in and be judged by. However, bodybuilding is a sport that encompasses one's whole life; it is an opportunity for business prospects and personal growth; it has the ability to impact relationships and all other aspects of one's life. To decide to be humble and not talk about your success and not promote yourself as someone who has done great things with your body as a result of dedication and hard work is to damage your ambition and career and to welcome underachievement and shortcomings. It is to invite low levels of satisfaction, all for what? To appease those who desire the opportunity to see a bodybuilder who is humble and quiet?

There are many ways to be outgoing and create wonderful opportunities without being arrogant and self-absorbed and without being perceived that way. It is confidence, quiet or loud, that demands attention and creates opportunities. It is admirable to be humble in a way that still displays confidence. It is refreshing to see a bodybuilder who is not an egomaniac and completely self-absorbed and who is quietly confident in his or her abilities and accomplishments. Though it can be admirable and respectable to be a person of this nature and demeanor, I believe that the more out-going and forward-thinking bodybuilder will create more opportunities 9 out of 10 times. These are worthwhile opportunities because they can bring fulfillment, bring personal rewards, generate income, and increase influence. One can make so much more of a difference in the world by sharing success, than hiding success because success stories motivate and inspire others to do the same. Don't wait for opportunities to pass you by or show themselves; go out there and make them happen by being pro-active and confident in your abilities to contribute something based on your achievements.

The best advice I can give is to be yourself as often as possible and alter faulty behavior in order to further your career, be of great influence, and create more positive opportunities. If you're naturally a quiet, shy, and humble person, it will be much easier for you to behave in that way. Unfortunately in this industry you will likely excel more slowly, but that is just a result of the way this industry works and how a timid approach to life plays a part in that. Conversely, if you are naturally more out-going, out-spoken, and feel more comfortable in the spotlight, playing that role will be very easy, and you will likely get more opportunities solely based on your personality and character. Just as outgoing people are likely going to be better actors in drama or theater and more comfortable on stage with a microphone, they are also more likely to have more opportunities as bodybuilders because it is a sport that is designed to reward the people who make the most of it. I have seen this happen in my life many times, including recently when I represented Bodybuilding.com, the largest bodybuilding company in the world. I made an exceptional first impression and got invited back to work with them at the Olympia, the Super Bowl of bodybuilding. I wasn't humble, but rather, I was eccentric, outgoing, friendly, and interactive with a receptive community. I had a lot of fun taking charge at the booth, though I was the only non IFBB Professional athlete working the booth that weekend. Had I been a quiet and humble person behind the booth, there is no doubt in my mind that I would not have been invited back. It was purely a result of my outgoing demeanor and enthusiasm and confidence that I was rewarded the opportunity to work with the biggest bodybuilding company on the biggest stage later in the year. There are missed opportunities every time we think we need to act humble because that is what we believe a specific audience wants to see. Be extraordinary not overlooked.

I don't mean to say that you can't be successful as a quiet, humble, and respectful bodybuilder; there are many who are. I just don't want you to think that if you're naturally outgoing you need to curb your enthusiasm and behavior in order to live according to expectations that you perceive a non-bodybuilding community has for bodybuilders. Be yourself and don't sell yourself short. And if you do happen to be a quiet, humble vegan bodybuilder, consider the ramifications of not projecting yourself more. You are in no way doing animals a favor by being humble. Be comfortable as you are, but realize that if you are an outstanding vegan bodybuilder, you have an incredible opportunity to influence people and save lives. You have to ask yourself if it is worth it to stand back and be the quiet, humble bodybuilder who goes about his or her life with little influence. Or is it more worthwhile to stand up and stand for something and make your voice heard and your message known so that animals don't have to suffer because you will change the minds of those who currently see animals as food rather than friends? It may not be a popular opinion, but I consider it a disservice to animals for a vegan who has the ability to influence people in a positive way to not use that influence appropriately and responsibly. It is something to think about. Being humble because you think it's "cool" or because you don't want to be "one of them" is completely ineffective. Being humble can be down right insulting to veganism and to bodybuilding, and it can marginalize your career as a bodybuilder whether you are vegan or not. It's not going to get you anywhere with potential sponsors. In business and in marketing, sponsors always go for the people who are smiling, friendly, outgoing, confident, social, and those who draw others in with a magnetic personality. Consider that when you consider quietly trying to build a bodybuilding career.

Sure, I've been called cocky or arrogant a few times throughout my life, but even as out-going as I am, I've been called humble just as many times. I am very outgoing because I know animals are counting on me, and I know the difference it will make for me as a person, in my career, and in the industries and movements I am involved in and support. I always want to stand up for those who can't be heard. If that means being called cocky as I save animals lives then that is what I'll continue to be called, but at the end of the day I will know that I made the right decision. Actions often speak louder than words and taking action is what I do best. I want to be as productive as I can be with everything involving my vegan bodybuilding lifestyle. The best way that I know how to do that is to be myself, plus a slightly even more outgoing self to accomplish everything that I want to in this industry. It is completely and totally worth it to go the extra mile and be myself plus a little more. Ultimately, I view being humble to get recognized for the action of being humble as an extreme form of arrogance. Additional arrogance is something the bodybuilding industry can definitely do without.

As a result of my busy lifestyle and being the biggest promoter of the vegan bodybuilding movement and message, I was recently advised to take a moment to slow down and stop and smell the roses by a member of my vegan bodybuilding website who observed my hectic life through my website blog posts. I replied with the response, "I know how to enjoy life, but I also know that so many are counting on me to be able to enjoy their lives (animals). So I have to keep myself busy to make better lives for others, and that gives me fulfillment. That is greater than anything I could do for myself for my own enjoyment. To me, fulfillment is greater than enjoyment, though they can be experienced simultaneously, which I am learning how to do." This statement demonstrates the outgoing confidence coupled with humble motivations behind the actions. It is worth acknowledging that the two extremes can be present at the same time in the same person. When an individual acknowledges both characteristics and the individual can feel the humbleness behind their actions inside their heart but display them with out-going confidence to an audience, it is a highly powerful and influential combination that one can use to create change in the world.

4. Compete on stage; it is the best way to learn.

You can read all you want about competitive bodybuilding and study it thoroughly in great detail; you can train and lift weights and eat like a body-builder all you want, but there is no better lesson in bodybuilding than competing on stage first-hand. There is no adequate replacement for actually being a bodybuilder on stage going through quarter turns and mandatory poses in front of judges. I've said many times, "Until you get up on stage in posing trunks and compete, you don't know what it's like to be a bodybuilder." Bodybuilding is tough. The diet is tough; the training is tough; the prepara-tion is tough. But one of the toughest aspects of all is getting up on stage and holding poses for long periods of time. It is physically, mentally, and emo-tionally exhausting. To contract and hold every muscle possible for judges is an experience only competitive bodybuilders know. Posing in front of a mir-ror at home or with a posing coach, or even in a situation where you pretend that you are on stage, still can't duplicate the feeling and experience of actu-ally being on the bodybuilding stage in front of judges and a critical audience. Some joke that the toughest part is wearing the tiny posing trunks in front of friends, family, and strangers; but for me, that is the easy part. The tough part for me is knowing that every aspect of my physique is on display, and the flaws that others perceive are a direct correlation with the effort I put into my preparation. I don't want to let others down by participating in a competition ill prepared or with major flaws. As a perfectionist by nature, being on stage is the hardest part of competitive bodybuilding for me. Holding intense muscle contractions for prolonged periods is a close second.

Many aspiring bodybuilders will talk about their lives as bodybuilders and even call themselves bodybuilders because they follow most of the body-building lifestyle, but so many of them will never get on stage and never get to experience first-hand what it is to compete. The primary reason for this, as I have perceived it, is that many aspiring bodybuilders are waiting for the perfect moment, when they are at their very best; they are too intimidated to get up on stage at any other time. The risk involved in this approach is that they may never get on stage because there will always be an excuse. I hear all the time from others comments such as these: "I'm not big enough. I'm not ready. I don't have all the poses down yet. I don't have what it takes to get on stage. I couldn't possibly be competitive with the other bodybuilders. I would compete if it weren't for the pre-contest diet." The list goes on and on. I've said some of these things myself, and I've also said that one of my personal worries is not being totally prepared when getting up on stage; but by getting up on stage, I learn so much and can take what I've learned and improve.

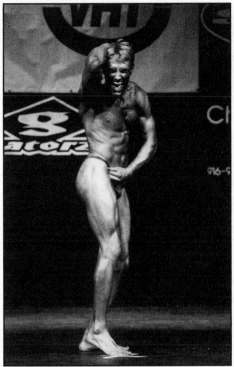

Robert placing 4th of 7 in his first competition in 2003

Though I had my hesitations at first (though fewer hesitations than most; I couldn't wait to get on stage), I finally decided to get on stage so the opportunity wouldn't pass me by. Sure, maybe I wasn't as ready as I could have been, and I could have spent a couple of additional years putting on more mass and size, but I really wanted to compete, and I did. In my first competition, I placed 4th of 7. My next time on stage found me in first place followed by a 2nd place finish, and my career took off from there. Even as time went on, I placed as low as last place and as high as 1st place for a second time. The fact is I kept after it, kept learning and kept improving. I just competed three times in the spring of 2009, and I placed in the top 5 in all three competitions including a 1st place finish at the 2009 INBA Northwestern USA Natural Bodybuilding Championships that were held in Portland, OR and a 3rd place finish at the 2009 NPC Bill Pearl High Desert Classic in Bend, OR (named after the great vegetarian bodybuilder who was voted the best physique in the world back in the '70s as a vegetarian athlete. He also beat Arnold Schwarzenegger on stage, as a vegetarian).

Robert with Arnold Schwarzennegger, 2001

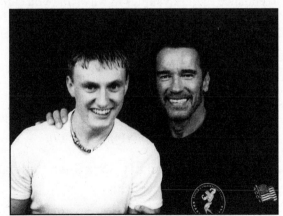

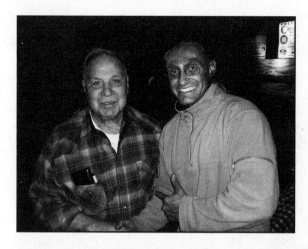

*Robert with Bill Pearl after
placing 3rd at the 2009 Bill
Pearl High Desert Classic*

There is no better way to learn than to put on a pair of posing trunks for men or a posing suit for women and get up there under the hot, bright lights in front of a live audience and give it your best effort. If you have ever thought about competing, I encourage you wholeheartedly to do so! Don't let this opportunity pass you by. You don't want to be asking yourself years down the road, "What might have been had I given competitive bodybuilding a shot?" Take action and make it happen. You'll likely find that competing is quite thrilling, a very powerful experience, and an inspiring act of self-confidence and self trust.

If you are a natural bodybuilder, meaning you haven't used any anabolic drugs like steroids or growth hormone, I suggest you begin by competing within the natural organizations so you can compete against other all natural athletes who will be drug tested at the show (usually polygraph test or urine test, sometimes both). That way, everyone is on the same level, and you can be competitive without going up against those who have used anabolic agents to enhance their physiques in ways that you can't match naturally.

Some of the natural bodybuilding organizations include the following:

International Natural Bodybuilding Federation (INBF) –
www.inbf.net

International Natural Bodybuilding Association (INBA) –
www.naturalbodybuilding.com

The Organization of Competitive Bodybuilders (OCB) –
www.theocbwebsite.com

There are even a few very small, independent natural bodybuilding organizations or promoters such as I AM Fitness by Rodney Hawthorne in Washington State:

(www.leaguelineup.com/welcome.asp?url=iamfitness)

There are other bodybuilding organizations as well including the most popular bodybuilding organization, the National Physique Committee (NPC), www.npcnewsonline.com, which is an amateur division leading to the International Federation of Body Building and Fitness (IFBB), www.ifbb.com. The NPC has some "natural" shows as well, but my understanding is that only the winners are drug tested or there is random drug testing, so not all of the athletes are tested. However, the natural bodybuilding organizations hold competitions where every bodybuilder is accurately tested for drug use within the past five to seven years.

The natural organizations have professional divisions within their organizations as well, so it is possible to be a professional natural bodybuilder and compete for prize money. However, the prize money is much smaller in comparison to the prize money offered for professional unnatural bodybuilders within the IFBB. A natural bodybuilding champion at the professional level may win $1,000 to $5,000 at a competition. An IFBB professional bodybuilding champion may win $10,000 to $150,000 for a first place finish, by comparison. Regardless of the type of bodybuilding, natural or unnatural, most of the income made by the athletes is through sponsorship. Some companies such as BSN and MuscleTech have been known to pay bodybuilders seven-figure salaries and high six-figure salaries to represent their product lines.

Review the websites listed above to find contests in your region. Start with a local competition where your friends, family, trainers, peers, and others you know may be able to attend and support you. It is often helpful to have people you know in the audience to help give you support and shout posing instructions to you since you don't have a mirror to look at. It is also helpful to have someone you know backstage to help you with your tan application, pump-up, and keep you calm as you prepare to get out on stage. Having friends cheer for you is always a helpful bonus.

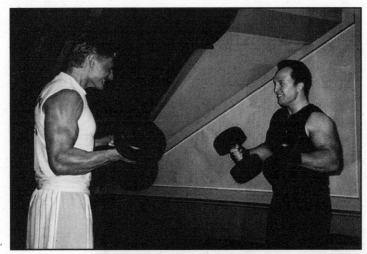

Robert with friend Leonard Bakulo training on board a cruise ship, 2002

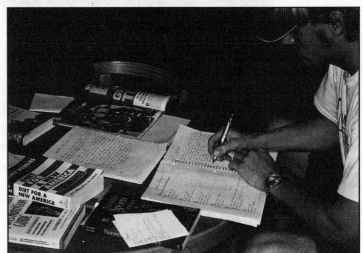

Working on a cruise ship in 2003, Robert is determined to get his writing career off the ground

5. Work harder than anyone else you know

So often we find reasons to give up, make excuses why we never reached our full potential, and find explanations for our shortcomings. This behavior can be directly related to our work ethic.

I wrote an article called True Intensity that is featured in my book *Your Personal Best* and is on my vegan bodybuilding website. It is one of my signature hardcore articles. You can visit my veganbodybuilding.com website to read it, but for this book I wanted to write a new article dedicated to work ethic:

Increase Your Work Ethic to Create Your Own Results
By Robert Cheeke
June 23, 2009

I believe the term "hard work" gets thrown around way too loosely and way too carelessly in our society. Every day people walk around describing "hard work" as if they actually think they have some sort of comprehension of what that means. Every day people think that working 40 hours a week is "hard" and that creating time in their schedule to peel themselves away from the television or their TV dinner to exercise is "hard work." The truth is, most people in our culture have no idea what it means to work hard or to believe in something so much that they'll dedicate their life to it and do what it takes to accomplish it. Most people don't truly commit to something that is exceptional or outstanding and work excruciatingly hard at it every day. Most people simply don't have it in them. You can blame it on society; you can blame it on culture; you can blame it on lifestyle and conveniences or traditions; but I choose to blame it on the individual. Average people don't work hard unless they are forced to by necessity. It takes effort, work, and time, and most people are not interested in investing any of those things as long as they have their 40-hour per week jobs, television programs, fast food, and partner or family to share this time with. Average people don't want to change anymore than they have to because they've put in their eight hours for the day and they're ready to kick back, rest their feet, and relax. Sure, people still complain that they don't have enough money to pay bills, improve healthcare, support their children better, enhance their lifestyles, and bring more fulfillment to their lives; but they're not willing to work hard to change. It's just too much to ask. Average people would rather become obese or get sick before they'd ever think about starting an exercise program, following a sound nutrition program, or applying themselves more in areas such as work or relationships.

What makes me any different? The only thing that makes me any different than anyone else in this society when it comes to hard work is the fact that I am aware of how lazy we are and I've chosen to do something about it. That's it. That's the only thing that separates me and other hard-working people from those who don't work hard in our society. We simply took the time to acknowledge it and conclude that being lazy isn't the right thing to do, that there is so much more to life than just getting by. We realized that the world is a wonderful place with endless opportunities to succeed and to contribute in monumental ways, and we concluded that the road to success is paved in hard work day in and day out in all aspects of life. We also came to the realization that hard work doesn't mean boring or unfulfilling work. Some of the greatest times of my life resulted from working harder than anyone else and putting in 15-hour days doing truly meaningful things in my life. We're also fully aware that there are plenty of people in all parts of the world who work way harder than we do and don't have the privileges we have, the opportunities we have, the tools and resources that we have, or the support that we have. Billions work from dawn to dusk to simply survive; others seem to not even try; others work hard to thrive. Where do you fall among these groups?

The first step in embracing a new work ethic is to let go of ego and accept the fact that you really don't work very hard. When I came to the conclusion that I was lazy, selfish, had poor time management, made bad decisions, and didn't care very much about what I was doing, I realized I was just like everyone else and I needed to make a change immediately. I made a change and became successful immediately, found immediate meaning in the hard work I was doing, and found it to be enjoyable, fulfilling, and rewarding. Most of us just aren't willing to work any harder than we are now. If we can change our way of thinking to understand how to work hard and understand why it is important to work hard, we can do incredible things with our lives and that is what life should be about.

Here are some tips to improve your work ethic:

- Get rid of your television. It distracts you from doing productive and meaningful things in your life and eats up an incredible amount of time.
- Determine what you love to do the most and spend more time doing it.
- Find true meaning in your life and pursue it with passion.
- Reduce the time you spend on the Internet.
- Observe the work ethic of the people who are the most successful in any given industry.
- Observe the work ethic of those who rely on their work ethic to survive.
- Learn how to manage your time effectively and efficiently.
- Set specific work ethic goals.
- Understand how investment of effort leads directly to the attainment of goals.
- Really believe in what it is you are doing. Belief will automatically improve motivation and work ethic.

Robert's Recap of the Most Important lessons to be learned and followed in Bodybuilding

When you keep a journal to track all of your training and nutrition programs as well as notes about how your life is going in general, it gives you added tools to use when evaluating your bodybuilding lifestyle. When you are consistent as a result of keeping record of your bodybuilding life, you get real results, you improve, and you enjoy the bodybuilding lifestyle. When you succeed as a result of how consistent you are and how much fun you're having, don't sell yourself short by being too humble just because you think that is what people expect from you or because you think you have some obligation to humility. Often it is the quiet, humble people who are left behind when opportunities present themselves. When you're ready to compete, the best way to learn is by getting up on stage. You can practice all you want, but until you've been under the bright lights in a pair of posing trunks or posing suit in front of an audience and judges, you don't know what it's like to be a competitive bodybuilder. When you put everything together and then resolve to work harder than anyone you know, you will be set on a road that few get to travel down. You'll succeed and create your own opportunities to get sponsored, to get jobs, to build opportunities for success in areas of passion or interest, and you'll enjoy life in amazing ways. You'll be respected for your work ethic, and you'll inspire other people to demand more from themselves, which creates a better life for them and in turn contributes to the causes they support.

Robert's Top 10 tips for incorporating the most important lessons to be learned and followed in bodybuilding

1. Be a doer not a talker. Jump inside the action and do the things necessary to learn how to be the best bodybuilder you can be.

2. Hold yourself accountable and thrive in that environment. Be known for your follow-through and your ability to complete tasks including getting to the gym regularly, eating consistently, and supplementing when necessary.

3. Learn when to be humble and when to be yourself. When you are yourself and act naturally with all your enthusiasm around your sport and success you've had in it, you'll likely be a natural spokesperson for the industry.

4. When people tell you that you can't do something, show them you can do it, and make a living out of proving people wrong.

5. Compete on stage because it builds character, builds your résumé, gives you more credibility, and gives you another component to your weight lifting and bodybuilding program.

6. Work exceptionally hard and make it evident to those around you. Some of the greatest role models in any industry, from any culture, from any generation, were people who worked excruciatingly hard and led by the example they set.

7. Learn from your mistakes. Don't let mistakes happen and be forgotten. Use every opportunity you can to learn from past mistakes.

8. Learn from your success. Don't let success go to your head without proper acknowledgement of how you got to that point in the first place.

9. Become a role model for people in your industry and work everyday as if they are watching your every move.

10. Don't give up. Don't ever give up on your dreams.

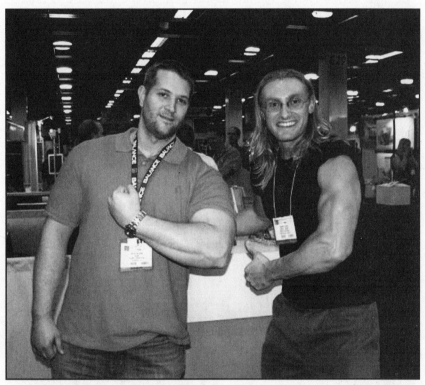

Robert with vegan power lifter and owner of Vegan Essentials, Ryan Wilson

"Robert Cheeke sparked my interest in vegan fitness and natural bodybuilding; before I first read an article about him, I thought that all bodybuilders used steroids and animal products. He also helped me find the strength to go vegan after half a decade of being a vegetarian. His example shattered the false ideas that I had been told all of my life about veganism, especially in regard to health and bodybuilding. Robert is living proof that you can be a champion bodybuilder on an ethical and healthful vegan diet. No longer do we need to reference the silverback gorilla as an example of size and strength on a plant-based diet, because now we have Robert Cheeke!"

Dave Bishea
Writer, Student, Fan of Vegan Bodybuilding & Fitness,
Aspiring Vegan Bodybuilder
Houston, TX

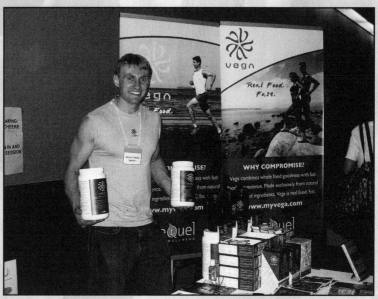

Working for Vega in 2005 in Canada

Chapter 6

Where Do You Get Your Protein?

"When I tell people that I'm vegan, the first question asked is, 'How do you get enough protein?' This immediately tells me that the person knows little or nothing about nutrition."

Robert Cheeke, Author

When people learn that I am a vegan bodybuilder, the most frequently asked question is, "Where do you get your protein?" I have been answering this question for nearly 15 years. It never gets any less annoying and will never go away as long as I am vegan and vocal about it—which will be forever, by the way. I accept that and understand that. Truth be told, I am excited to have a book that has an entire chapter dedicated to this topic, so I won't have to answer the question verbally anymore. I can just say, "It's all in my book and explained in detail. I suggest you give it a read. It will answer your question sufficiently." Having this book is a good tool for all of you as well, and I am sure you get asked the same question more often than any other question when it comes to your vegan lifestyle. Therefore, this resource should be helpful when addressing this extremely common question.

Before answering this question, we should consider why this question is being asked in the first place and determine our method of reply. What is the person trying to learn by proposing this question? Is it a sincere question or one asked for another reason?

To vegans, the question is silly. Vegans know there are plenty of plant-based foods packed with adequate and complete proteins. But care should be taken when answering the question. It would be harmful to the vegan cause to answer rudely or condescendingly. Some people are asking sincerely to truly learn because they innocently don't know better. Others may be asking because they want to know which are the preferred sources, so they can get ideas to incorporate into their diets. When the question is answered rudely and not with a lot of thought or tact, people receiving the answer will have a negative reaction and a negative impression of veganism, especially if their question was from sincere curiosity and desire to learn. We have to handle ourselves appropriately because it could lead to very positive discourse or very negative discourse, each of which has implications, and we want to do what is best for ourselves and our movement as often as possible.

Vegan bodybuilders who are frequently asked this question can lead by positive example to answer the protein question to the vegan and non-vegan communities. Even though we don't always think so at first, this common question can be legitimate without any ill intentions or attitude attached to it. Some people are sincerely looking for answers to learn more and to add more variety into their diet. And many others are asking because they know someone who is vegan and they are seeking out additional information to share with a friend or loved one.

Though I am annoyed by the question because it is a question that comes from ignorance, I do answer the question as respectfully as I can, and I tailor my response to the person asking the question. If I can tell that someone is being deliberately provocative and trying to lure me into an argument or debate or waiting for me to make a fool of myself, I will politely direct them to my websites, my documentaries, or to this book to get their question answered. I let them know there are meal programs and lists and charts and information that they will find interesting.

When you look like an athlete or a bodybuilder, you display to an audience that you clearly get enough protein in your diet. As a result, you may not have to address the question as often. Or people could be so surprised by a muscular physique built on a plant-based diet that they want to know more and more about it and how they can do it too. When you have a physique that speaks for itself, answering the question is easy. You can get away with listing off some common sources of plant protein, a few favorite meals, and add that training and dedication go along with it. It gives a quick, well-rounded answer that is often sufficient for the questioner.

Whatever method you choose to use when answering the protein question, proceed with confidence. You are always welcome to reference me, my websites, my documentaries, or my books; and you can encourage people to learn about a variety of vegan athletes who are out there everyday working hard to live a healthy active vegan lifestyle. I enjoy leading by example to take the burden off of other people. I use my physique to challenge common ways of thinking and to present new ways of thinking and understanding. Use your resources, including this resource, and feel comfortable in your discourse with others regarding this topic. If you struggle with your communication, look to those who have been doing it for a long time like the people who work for Vegan Outreach (www.veganoutreach.org) or other animal rights organizations that focus on positive conversations with others about various topics including protein intake on a vegan diet. My friend Nettie Schwager articulates this topic well in conversations and in countless letters to newspapers. Search for her work online for additional helpful resources.

Here is a list of some of the ways I have handled and addressed the protein question. After more than a decade of experience addressing this issue, the following list is ten examples of how I have responded to this question.

The Question: "Where do you get your protein?"

My response #1

"Protein is found in nearly every food and in higher amounts in certain foods like nuts, grains, beans, legumes, green vegetables, and in foods like tofu, tempeh, and in the form of protein powders and bars commonly made of up hemp, pea, rice, buckwheat, or soy protein. Eating a wide variety of foods makes it easy to get adequate protein from plant sources, and I eat a lot of heavy foods like burritos, sandwiches, wraps, almond butter, and grains like quinoa and brown rice. I also use protein powders and protein bars since I'm a bodybuilder and want extra protein, especially post-workout. Overall, I get most of my protein from eating a variety of food, just like everyone else."

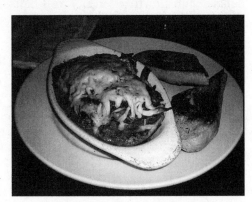

Vegan Lasagna from Ethos Vegan Kitchen – Orlando, FL

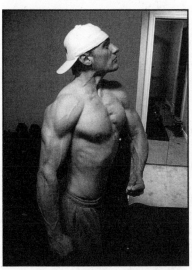

Photo by George Wong

My response #2

"I ingest more protein than almost anyone I know because I make it a point to do so. I eat six to eight meals a day, consuming a wide variety of foods, and I rack up about 300 grams of protein per day."

My response #3

"I don't rely on one main source of protein. Instead, I focus on various quality sources and get a broad spectrum of amino acids. I don't just rely on soy, but I eat some soy-based foods and focus primarily on plant-based whole foods. Some of my favorite foods are quinoa, kale, spinach, all types of beans, hemp, almonds, walnuts, peanut butter, tofu, tempeh, and protein drinks like Vega, which is made of hemp, pea, and rice protein. I also eat a bunch of different protein bars as snacks. In general, I make sure I eat as much color and variety as I can throughout the day. That way, I get plenty of protein."

My response #4

"Where do you get *your* protein? How do you monitor your cholesterol intake?"

My response #5

"I eat a wide variety of foods, and protein is one of the easiest components of nutrition to get in any well-balanced diet."

My response #6

"Do you know anyone with a protein deficiency?"

My response #7

"I have gained 70 pounds (enter your own results here) on a plant-based diet, so getting enough protein has never been an issue for me."

My response #8

"There is a great list of high protein foods on veganbodybuilding.com. The website lists the foods and their protein content so you can check out that resource to find out what types of foods vegans eat, including the highest protein foods. There are meal programs on the website as well as athlete bios so it should be really helpful and provide a lot of information regarding protein intake on a vegan diet. We have female and male athletes including 270-pound strong men, fitness models, professional athletes, and personal trainers who are all long-time vegans profiled on our website too. Check it out to see a variety of vegan athletes and learn about what we eat."

My response #9

"I just wrote a 300-page book (Champion Vegan Bodybuilder Robert Cheeke just wrote a 300-page book) all about vegan bodybuilding and there is an entire chapter dedicated to the protein issue on a vegan diet. The book includes more than 50 meal programs covering high protein meals and mass-building meal programs and should be an excellent resource to answer your question in detail. It's called *Vegan Bodybuilding & Fitness – The Complete Guide to Building Your Body on a Plant-Based Diet*. Check it out on www.veganbodybuildingbook.com."

My response #10

I just flex for them and say something in a playful manner like "Getting enough protein has never been a problem for me, and I eat more protein than almost anyone I know."

As much as I defend protein consumption for myself and for vegans in general, I have to say, in all honesty that most vegans I know probably don't get enough protein in their diets on a daily basis to maintain a healthy-looking build. I believe most vegan "athletes" do get enough protein because they are more conscious of it and make more of an effort to get adequate protein to assist their athletic performance. But when it comes to the general vegan population, I have to admit that most look as if they are on a low-protein consumption diet. I believe this happens for the same reason our general population is obese. Most people just don't pay attention to proper nutrition or just don't care enough to eat the best types of foods. Often times the vegan's focus is on activism, outreach, or political topics, and their own health isn't a priority. However, health should be a very high priority because the everyday vegan would be a much better activist if he or she spent more time focused on being healthy and being a very well-rounded effective activist. Eating well—getting enough protein and calories—and and being active and fit allows one to have more energy, be more convincing in health discussions with others and enables one to be more effective and more efficient in every-thing one does, simply by being healthier.

To be truly effective in your cause, you should stand out from the non-vegan population. An obese, sickly, or malnourished body is no different from the status quo. If you are truly passionate about the vegan movement, the first step is to stand out in a positive, healthy way. And that starts with caring about nutrition.

I know some of you are thinking, "Robert, that is easy for you to say because you are a vegan bodybuilder that many people look up to so you don't have to struggle with body image, weight gain, or weight loss and don't struggle with overall health on a vegan diet." I am always quick to respond to that suggestive statement by explaining to readers that I was 120 pounds when I became vegan in high school. Initially, I was a poor physical representative of the movement in regards to what the vegan stereotype image is. I weighed 155 pounds when I was a runner in college at Oregon State University for the track club and still wasn't the pinnacle of health. I wasn't always a muscular person; in fact, I never was. I was always small and scrawny before I was vegan and after I was vegan for many years, but it was never an issue, scapegoat, or area of blame until I was vegan. Was it fair? No. It's not fair, but I represented what people expected of me, which was to be another skinny vegan. And that is precisely what I was. I became a vegan bodybuilder out of personal interest, something I always wanted to do since I was a kid. I also did it to make a statement and effectively stand for something meaningful in my life. Just as my skinny physique was blamed on my veganism—even though in my case it didn't have anything to do with it since I was already skinny throughout my whole life—my muscle gains and my success as a bodybuilder were attributed to my vegan lifestyle. Is that fair? Not necessarily. Just as veganism was blamed for my skinny physique, veganism takes credit for my muscular physique; really, it was my hard-nosed determination, work ethic, and ability to demand excellence from myself that made the difference.

I would like to believe that my vegan diet helped inspire my muscle gains and physique transformation; but the truth is, with the amount of effort, training, and dedication I had for bodybuilding and transforming my physique, basically any diet would have worked. The vegan diet gets to take credit for this body transformation just as it is to blame for so many of us who represent the common stereotype of a weakling. It's not always fair, but it's how we're perceived, and we don't always get the opportunity to talk with people to explain ourselves. Most of our visibility is from afar. People see us from a distance and form an opinion about us. Non-verbal communication clearly outweighs verbal communication in its ability to influence ideas, opinions, and perceptions. How we carry ourselves and present ourselves non-verbally is of very high importance in the future success of our vegan movement.

When you are fit or muscular representatives of the vegan lifestyle, you open up doors for others who maybe had an interest in vegansim but feared they could never be strong on that diet until they spotted you and learned from your example. That is a pretty powerful position to be in to further the movement.

In summary, I think vegans can be better activists and make more of a difference simply by focusing more on being healthy. Then we get veganism to become synonymous with health and vitality and present a positive image to the general public. Let's counter the stereotype that associates veganism with inadequate protein intake and a sickly constitution.

I am including high protein meal programs as well as lists of high-protein foods to give you some ideas of ways to increase your protein intake.

High Protein Meal Programs based on six meals per day

<u>High Protein Meal Program #1</u>

Meal #1
> Protein smoothie with greens, fruit, hemp, pea, and rice protein (Vega)
> Protein bar
> 2 pieces of whole fruit
> 16 ounces of water

Meal #2
> Vega meal replacement drink
> Pita bread and hummus
> Cup of lentil soup
> 16 ounces of water

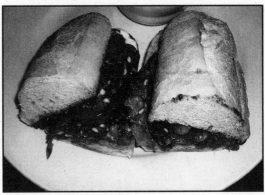

What's the Dilly Philly? Sandwich from Ethos Vegan Kitchen – Orlando, FL

Meal #3
2 tofu sandwiches with avocado, romaine lettuce, tomato
Protein smoothie
16 ounces of water

Meal #4
2 protein bars
2 pieces of whole fruit
16 ounces of water

Meal #5
Large bowl of buckwheat pasta with Vega omega 3-6-9 EFA oil
Large green salad with hemp seeds
Strips of baked tofu or tempeh with dipping sauce
Vega meal replacement drink
16 ounces of water

Meal 6
2 servings of walnuts
Vega protein pudding
2 slices of bread with almond butter
10 ounces of hemp milk

Estimated Totals:
Total Calories = 6,000
Total grams protein = 360g
Total grams of carbohydrates = 800g
Total grams of fats = 150g
Total water consumption = 128 ounces (factoring in water for
        protein drinks too)

High Protein Meal Program #2

Meal #1
Protein drink
Peanut butter and jam sandwich
2 non-dairy yogurts
2 pieces of fruit
16 ounces of water

Meal #2
Organic Food "Protein" Bar
PROBAR
Fruit smoothie
16 ounces of water

Meal #3
Large burrito
Green salad with hemp seeds and flax seeds and a variety of greens
10 ounce hemp milk
16 ounces of water

Meal #4
Bowl of lentil soup
Protein drink
Vega Vibrancy bar
16 ounces of water

Meal#5
Baked potato with beans, tofu, and broccoli
Green salad
16 ounces of water

Meal #6
Protein drink
2 pieces of fruit

Estimated Totals:
Total Calories = 5,400
Total grams protein = 285g
Total grams of carbohydrates = 815g
Total grams of fats = 110g
Total water consumption = 128 ounces (factoring in water for protein drinks too)

High Protein Meal Program #3

Meal #1
> 2 pancakes
> Plate of tofu scramble with tofu and vegetables and seasonings
> 16 ounce orange juice
> 16 ounces of water

Meal #2
> Vega meal replacement drink
> Protein bar
> 3 pieces of fruit
> 16 ounces of water

Meal #3
> 2 Tempeh Reuben sandwiches
> Green protein smoothie
> 16 ounces of water

Meal #4
> Protein bar
> 2 servings of assorted nuts
> 2 pieces of fruit
> 16 ounces of water

Meal #5
> Large bowl of quinoa, beans, kale, and tempeh
> Green salad with Vega omega 3-6-9 EFA oil
> 16 ounces of water

Meal #6
> Protein drink
> 2 pieces of fruit

Estimated Totals:

> Total Calories = 5,800
> Total grams protein = 270g
> Total grams of carbohydrates = 865g
> Total grams of fats = 140g
> Total water consumption = 116 ounces (factoring in water for
> protein drinks too)

In addition to the previously suggested methods of answering the question, "Where do you get your protein?" you can use the article below to provide an answer.

This article has found its way into full-multi-page spreads in magazines such as *Beyond Fitness Magazine* and *Organic Lifestyle Magazine*. It answers the question about where I get my protein as a vegan athlete and brings to light the fact that vegan bodybuilding doesn't have to be considered an "oxymoron." Feel free to use this article from this book or from my website to share with others. Re-post it on your website and share it with your social media communities.

Vegan Bodybuilding is NOT an Oxymoron
by Robert Cheeke, Vegan Bodybuilder - January 7, 2007

If there is a question vegans hear more than any other, it is, "How do you get your protein?" I often respond by asking the individual if they know anyone with a protein deficiency. Protein is found in nearly all foods and they are abundant in seeds, nuts, legumes, vegetables, and other plant-based foods.

In North America, we are taught from a young age to believe that the only good sources of protein come from animals. This is simply not true. In fact, it is proven by scores of scientific studies that plant-based sources of protein are easier for the human body to digest and absorb. Plus, plant-based foods do not come with many of the negative health implications associated with a diet rich in animal protein such as high cholesterol, high blood pressure, and cardiovascular disease.

Another advantage of plant-based foods is that they help promote an alkaline environment in the body. All animal protein is acid-forming, whereas most plant protein is alkaline forming. Essentially, an alkaline diet is the exact opposite of the high protein, high fat, low carb diets that have recently been in vogue. Because our body's ideal pH is slightly alkaline, our diets should reflect this and also be slightly alkaline. A diet high in acidic foods such as animal protein, sugar, caffeine, and processed foods tends to deplete the body of alkaline minerals such as calcium, magnesium, and potassium, making us more susceptible to chronic and degenerative disease.

Though a vegan diet is often a topic of concern when it comes to athletic performance, those concerns are unwarranted. As a vegan bodybuilder, I compete in a sport dominated by meat eaters, most of whom scoff at the idea that one could get sufficient protein from plants to be competitive. I do not consume any animal products whatsoever, not even dairy or eggs. Instead, I focus on eating a wide variety of plant-based whole foods. My protein comes primarily from hemp, tofu, tempeh, beans, nuts, seeds, grains, rice, fruits, and vegetables. By getting my protein from a wide variety of sources, I am ensuring my body receives a balance of essential amino acids.

Though I try to get as much protein as possible from whole foods, I often supplement with plant-based protein powders to help me meet my target of 1.5g of protein per pound of bodyweight for building muscle mass. My favorite protein powder source is hemp. In addition to being rich in complete protein, it is also a great source of essential fatty acids, antioxidants, vitamins, minerals, fiber, and chlorophyll.

Hemp protein is a quality source of arginine, histidine, methionine, and cysteine and also contains all the branched-chain amino acids crucial for repair and growth of lean body mass. Furthermore, almost two-thirds of hemp protein is comprised of edestin, a protein found only in hemp and the form of protein most similar to that of the human body. Hemp protein is also very easily digested and assimilated, making it one of the finest sources of protein in the plant kingdom.

Other great commonly available plant-based protein powders include yellow pea, brown rice, and soy. Though soy protein has been a staple in my diet for years, I have recently reduced my consumption of it because I am concerned about developing food sensitivities and/or allergies. Too much of a good thing can be detrimental to overall health, and my feeling is that soy is becoming overly pervasive in vegan and vegetarian diets. There are so many good alternatives such as hemp, pea, rice, and flax that I feel I don't need to rely on just soy protein powder anymore.

When I am on the run and don't have time to prepare a meal, I take a complete plant-based whole food meal replacement called Vega. Formulated by Brendan Brazier, a professional Ironman triathlete and fellow vegan, Vega is a quick and easy way for me to get quality nutrition. It contains many of my favorite foods, including hemp, pea, flax, rice, chlorella, and maca; and I especially like the fact that it contains five sources of quality protein, ensuring a balanced array of essential amino acids. I also snack on Vega energy bars before and after workouts for an extra boost.

Keep in mind that a high protein diet can be taxing on the liver and kidneys so it is important to drink a lot of water (I personally drink over a gallon a day as often as possible) to help the body's organs process the large amounts of protein. The great thing about plant protein is that it is much easier to digest and assimilate than animal protein, making the body's job easier and providing a greater nutritional yield. I also recommend eating smaller meals more frequently to ensure your muscles will always be fueled and nourished, providing the best opportunity for recovery, growth, and achieving your desired results.

As a vegan bodybuilder, I want to show others that it is possible to gain significant muscle and strength on a vegan diet, and I want to inspire others to follow this lifestyle. I love being vegan and knowing that I am having a positive impact on our society and culture. I believe that a plant-based diet is one of the best things you can do for your health and the well-being of our environment.

Robert Cheeke is a competitive bodybuilder and the 2005 INBA Northwestern USA Natural Bodybuilding Overall Novice Champion. He is also President and founder of Vegan Bodybuilding & Fitness, a company dedicated to supporting natural vegan bodybuilders and fitness enthusiasts (www.veganbodybuilding.com).

List of High Protein Foods:

The following chart shows the amount of protein in various vegan foods and also the number of grams of protein per 100 calories. To meet protein recommendations, the typical adult male vegan needs only 2.2 to 2.7 grams of protein per 100 calories, and the typical adult female vegan needs only 2.3 to 2.9 grams of protein per 100 calories. These recommendations can be easily met from vegan sources. Those numbers are easy targets for anyone. Bodybuilders should focus on 1-2 grams of protein per pound of bodyweight to maintain muscle and make muscle-building gains.

Protein Content of Selected Vegan Foods

Food	Amount	Protein (gm)	Protein (gm/100 cal)
Tempeh	1 cup	31	9.5
Seitan	4 ounces	15-31	21.4-22.1
Soybeans, cooked	1 cup	29	9.6
Veggie dog	1 link	8-26	13.3-20
Veggie burger	1 patty	5-24	3.8-21.8
Lentils, cooked	1 cup	18	7.8
Tofu, firm	4 ounces	8-15	10-12.2
Kidney beans, cooked	1 cup	15	6.8
Lima beans, cooked	1 cup	15	6.8
Black beans, cooked	1 cup	15	6.3
Chickpeas, cooked	1 cup	15	5.4
Pinto beans, cooked	1 cup	14	6
Black-eyed peas, cooked	1 cup	13	6.7
Vegetarian baked beans	1 cup	12	5.2
Quinoa, cooked	1 cup	11	3.5
Soymilk, commercial, plain	1 cup	3-10	3-12
Tofu, regular	4 ounces	2-10	2.3-10.7
Bagel	1 medium(3 oz)	9	3.7
Peas, cooked	1 cup	9	3.4
Textured Vegetable Protein (TVP), cooked	1/2 cup	8	8.4
Peanut butter	2 Tbsp.	8	4.1
Spaghetti, cooked	1 cup	7	3.4
Spinach, cooked	1 cup	6	11
Soy yogurt, plain	6 ounces	6	6
Bulgur, cooked	1 cup	6	3.7
Sunflower seeds	1/4 cup	6	3.3
Almonds	1/4 cup	6	2.8
Broccoli, cooked	1 cup	5	10.5
Whole wheat bread	2 slices	5	3.9
Cashews	1/4 cup	5	2.7
Almond butter	2 Tbsp	5	2.4
Brown rice, cooked	1 cup	5	2.1
Potato	1 medium(6 oz)	4	2.6

Sources: USDA Nutrient Database for Standard Reference, Release 12, 1998 and manufacturers' information.

A list on http://www.veganbodybuilding.com/?page=article_ commonfoods will show you not only lists of high protein foods but also high-calcium foods, high-magnesium foods, high-iron foods, etc.

Robert's Recap of where to get your protein

As a vegan, there is no doubt you will be receiving the protein question for the rest of your life. Now you know a lot of responses to use and know different ways to handle this question and these situations. When asked where you get your protein, evaluate the person's sincerity and interest and decide how much time you want to invest in your answer. Protein is very easy to get for anyone, no matter what their diet is as long as they consume adequate and sufficient calories. Let your physique do the talking as a vegan bodybuilder or vegan athlete, and it will answer the question for you. If your physique isn't ready to answer the question, use logic, reason, and sensibility as you provide information for those asking the questions or simply direct them to this book or to my vegan bodybuilding website. I'll take it from there with pre-written material directed at this exact question of the unique whereabouts of protein that some people think eludes the plant-based diet, when in fact it is in abundance, like all other components of nutrition.

Robert's Top 10 tips for getting sufficient protein and dealing with the popular question we're all asked "Where do you get your Protein?"

1. Eat a lot of food, and more importantly, eat sufficient quantities of nutrient-dense foods to fuel your body and nourish your muscles after exercise.

2. Discover what the best sources of protein are; determine which of those foods are your favorites and incorporate them regularly. If you enjoy eating the high protein foods, it won't seem like a chore to do so.

3. Eat consistently throughout the day, every two to three hours, to ensure you keep your body in an anabolic state to support your bodybuilding efforts and to constantly nourish your body.

4. Learn more about protein and its function in the body and the role that it plays in bodybuilding. The more you learn about it, know about it, care about it, and the more attention you give it, the better you will be as a bodybuilder.

5. When asked about your protein consumption, answer the question with confidence. Give examples of some of your favorite protein sources, and point to references like this book and the vegan bodybuilding website, which provide additional information. Give examples of other vegan athletes as well, especially those in power sports, not just endurance vegan athletes.

6. Get your blood tested so you can check your creatinine levels and find out if you're on the low end of protein consumption or the high end based on your age, gender, height, weight, and activity level. When you get your results, you can determine what adaptations or changes need to be made in your diet.

7. Create a protein target for yourself each day and physically write it down so you know the exact number of grams of protein you are trying to reach or exceed in any given day. Document your food intake and chart your progress. This will help you attain your daily goals.

8. Once you reach a specific protein level and your body adapts to it, gets bigger and stronger, and your weight increases, you can slowly increase your protein consumption as well to support your physical gains.

9. Conduct experiments on yourself with low, moderate, and high protein diets without changing anything in your exercise or sleep schedules. Evaluate how your body responds to various protein intakes for periods of 4-8 weeks and determine what quantity of protein works best for you based on your goals and how you feel.

10. Eat whole foods often because they are packed full of amino acids. Amino acids are the building blocks of protein and contribute greatly to your bodybuilding progression.

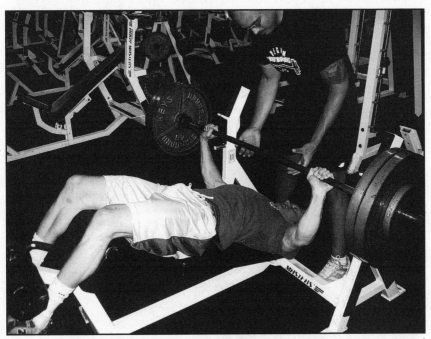

Robert lifting weights with friend Jeremy Moore spotting

"Robert Cheeke is one of my best friends. Robert has an energy that you rarely find in anyone. I've never met anyone able to take on their training 100% while still being able to handle taking on so many different aspects of the vegan movement 100% as well. There isn't a better person at multi-tasking in the world. Of course, having this type of personality you never only experience ups but also downs. The difference is that the downs never slow down Robert. He always keeps going with the same enthusiasm until his job is done."

Jeremy Moore
Professional Cyclist, Organic Athlete board member, friend
Pasadena, MD

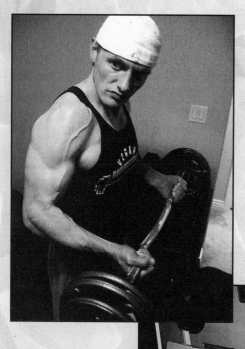

Training in Canada, 2006
(photo by George Wong)

Training at Loprinzi's Gym
Portland, OR 2009
(photo by Brian Van Peski)

Chapter 7

Choosing the Exercises that Yield the Best Results

"If you want to get big, you gotta learn to feel it. No exercise works if you don't feel it in the muscle that you're targeting. A lot of guys rely on mirrors to tell them whether or not an exercise is working, but that doesn't make sense to me. I think about getting the ultimate contraction in the muscle I'm targeting, and I don't stop until I feel that."

Jay Cutler
IFBB Pro Bodybuilder, 3-Time Mr. Olympia

Just like the idea that not all foods are created equally, the same can be said for exercises; some are inherently better than others. When we're talking about bodybuilding, some exercises stand out as being superior in many ways for good reasons. Most of us would agree that when it comes to aerobic fitness and improving endurance, running is superior to walking. It accomplishes the goal more efficiently, and adaptation and improvement come much more quickly. Methods of exercise and training can be compared in all sports, and superior exercises reveal themselves for their unique sport-specific interest and the benefits that they deliver.

When it comes to bodybuilding, the common understanding and belief is that multi-joint compound exercises are the best exercises to perform to gain muscle, strength, and overall size and muscle development. Within the compound exercises, there are favorites that stand alone among many bodybuilders and are considered the best. Some will go so far as to say that other exercises are not even necessary because the few compound exercises engage the entire body and do so in effective ways. Others will have a varied approach using a combination of compound exercises with isolation exercises, and others will have different approaches still. With all the different styles of training, one thing that appears to be a universal truth is that compound exercises simply are the best. If one has healthy joints, is injury-free, and can handle the stress, compound movements should be performed often as the primary exercises in a bodybuilding program.

When bodybuilders are asked to name the most effective exercises, the overwhelming majority name dead lifts, squats, and bench press. Some will go on to add power cleans, shoulder press, leg press, and occasionally some additional barbell and dumbbell exercises. I am a believer that these fundamental core exercises will indeed create a foundation of strength and power and will yield positive results in muscle gain and progression in bodybuilding. I am a firm believer that these core exercises are superior to other exercises, and a healthy person should perform these in order to get the most out of their workouts.

But what if you're not a healthy person because you have injuries in the lower back, shoulder, knee, or other joint? What if you can't do squats because of a weak back or bad knees? What if you can't perform overhead presses because of a pinched nerve or a shoulder that goes in and out of placement regularly? Well, that is when training adaptations need to be made; substitute exercises are utilized and become mainstays. I know this scenario all too well. As a long-time fan of squats and dead lifts, I have had to take both powerful movements out of my workout routine entirely because of injury. I'm still a supporter of dead lifts and squats–the two most superior exercises for bodybuilding; but I am unable to perform them for myself because of a weak and vulnerable lower back that completely inhibits the movements and causes severe pain and trauma to the area when attempted.

I loved doing squats and was well on my way to a big and strong physique when I collapsed under the barbell and was crushed under nearly 300 pounds when I was 21 years old preparing for a bodybuilding competition. My spine has never been the same, and I have had to make adaptations. Though I can't perform squats because of the stress it puts on my lower back and the injuries it causes because of a specific rotation in my tail bone, I can perform heavy leg presses and have pressed over 900 pounds on a number of occasions. I can no longer do dead lifts either because of the curvature of my lower spine and the pressure it puts on my nerves and nerve tendons. However, there are back exercises I can do that support my upper body and allow me to pull heavy amounts of weight such as T-bar rows and variations of bent-over rows. I fully understand that T-bar rows and bent-over rows can't replace dead lifts, but in my case, they are an adaptation that I embrace because they still allow me to lift heavy weights with my back. I can still move heavy weights on back exercises and I still win competitions even with limitations on specific power exercises I can do. I push myself to the limit no matter what exercise I'm doing, so I find ways to hammer my back with everything from rows to sets of 30 pull-ups or heavy-weighted pull-ups to challenge me to new levels of intensity, even if I can no longer do my former favorite exercises pulling hundreds of pounds. Even without squats in my bodybuilding training routine, my legs are my most dominant muscle group when I compete on stage. I learned that if you want success bad enough, you'll find a way to get there even if you have to take a road less traveled and are forced to be creative in your exercise selection.

If you are able to do the best exercises that you can to bring out the best in your physique, I encourage you to do so, but proceed with caution. There is nothing worse than seeing a highly motivated person with lots of potential get hurt doing a simple exercise and get sidelined, taken out of a sport they love as a result. This, as you can imagine, can have an incredible downward-spiral effect on the entire life of a person who has so much passion for exercise. All of a sudden, everything in life becomes less enjoyable to a person who has to sit back and not participate in one of their life's passions. So please, tread softly and with caution and care. It pays to be safe in the world of bodybuilding. Squats, dead lifts, and other compound movements aren't anything to mess around with. Learn how to do the exercises correctly before doing them regularly. My career completely changed as a result of two extremely painful injuries to my lower back involving those two power exercises with hundreds of pounds that I still feel residual painful effects from today. I have found ways to overcome them and move forward with replacement exercises, but the injuries put major dents in the progress of my bodybuilding career and still have an impact on it today, limiting some of my abilities to reach my fullest potential. My back hasn't fully recovered from those injuries. They still flare up in ways so severe that sometimes I'm unable to walk and have had to make emergency phone calls to doctors to fix my situation. This is my life now as a result of injuries. I still win bodybuilding competitions, still make it on the cover of magazines, and still live a fulfilling life; but I always wonder what might have been had I not hurt myself so dramatically that it impacts my career every ensuing year. Be careful. Trust me; I know how much it hurts to get injured and have life change as a result.

Based on your own bodybuilding goals, you'll want to select the best exercises for you. In general, compound exercises and free-weight exercises seem to be the most popular and proven for creating positive results. Be careful; be safe; learn how to do the exercises right. Always warm-up sufficiently before engaging in any of the power compound exercises. If you're injured, do not attempt any of the power exercises.

The following is an excerpt from an article on strengthening exercises. It breaks down various types of exercise and explains the role each type plays in an exercise or bodybuilding weight training program.

Strengthening exercise

Strengthening exercise increases muscle strength and mass, bone strength, and the body's metabolism. It can help attain and maintain proper weight and improve body image and self-esteem. A certain level of muscle strength is needed to do daily activities, such as walking, running and climbing stairs. Strengthening exercises increase this muscle strength by putting more strain on a muscle than it is normally accustomed to receiving. This increased load stimulates the growth of proteins inside each muscle cell that allow the muscle as a whole to contract. There is evidence indicating that strength training may be better than aerobic exercise alone for improving self-esteem and body image. Weight training allows one immediate feedback, through observation of progress in muscle growth and improved muscle tone. Strengthening exercise can take the form of isometric, isotonic and iso-kinetic strengthening.

ISOMETRIC EXERCISE. During isometric exercises, muscles contract. However, there is no motion in the affected joints. The muscle fibers maintain a constant length throughout the entire contraction. The exercises are usually performed against an immovable surface or object such as pressing one's hand against a wall. The muscles of the arm are contracting but the wall is not reacting or moving as a result of the physical effort. Isometric training is effective for developing total strength of a particular muscle or group of muscles. It is often used for rehabilitation since the exact area of muscle weakness can be isolated and strengthening can be administered at the proper joint angle. This kind of training can provide a relatively quick and convenient method for overloading and strengthening muscles without any special equipment and with little chance of injury.

ISOTONIC EXERCISE. Isotonic exercise differs from isometric exercise in that there is movement of a joint during the muscle contraction. A classic example of an isotonic exercise is weight training with dumbbells and barbells. As the weight is lifted throughout the range of motion, the muscle shortens and lengthens. Calisthenics are also an example of isotonic exercise. These would include chin-ups, push-ups, and sit-ups, all of which use body weight as the resistance force.

ISOKINETIC EXERCISE. Isokinetic exercise utilizes machines that control the speed of contraction within the range of motion. Isokinetic exercise attempts to combine the best features of both isometrics and weight training. It provides muscular overload at a constant preset speed while a muscle mobilizes its force through the full range of motion. For example, an isokinetic stationary bicycle set at 90 revolutions per minute means that despite how hard and fast the exerciser works, the isokinetic properties of the bicycle will allow the exerciser to pedal only as fast as 90 revolutions per minute. Machines known as Cybex and Biodex provide isokinetic results; they are generally used by physical therapists and are not readily available to the general population.

Cardiac rehabilitation

Exercise can be very helpful in prevention and rehabilitation of cardiac disorders and disease. With an individually designed exercise program set at a level considered safe for that individual, people with symptoms of heart failure can substantially improve their fitness levels. The greatest benefit occurs as muscles improve the efficiency of their oxygen use, which reduces the need for the heart to pump as much blood. While such exercise doesn't appear to improve the condition of the heart itself, the increased fitness level reduces the total workload of the heart. The related increase in endurance should also translate into a generally more active lifestyle. Endurance or aerobic routines, such as running, brisk walking, cycling, or swimming, increase the strength and efficiency of the muscles of the heart.

— L. Fleming Fallon, Jr., MD, DrPH[7]

Robert ranks of Most Effective Bodybuilding Exercises

I will provide definitions and descriptions of each exercise taken from the Internet, but I also encourage you to search each exercise online to see what it looks like. You will find photos and videos of every exercise mentioned, and you'll learn how to do them properly. You can also ask a personal trainer at your gym or an experienced weight lifter or bodybuilder for tips on how to do these listed exercises properly.

Each exercise description has been extracted from an online definition of the exercise from www.answers.com. That website is able to eloquently de-

---

[7] http://www.answers.com/topic/exercise

scribe each exercise in detail and has proved to be an excellent resource for me. Each exercise is explained in easy-to-understand terms we can all mentally picture and then practice in the gym.

The following exercises are the best and should be performed if you're healthy and able for optimal results from your training program.

The Rankings - The Top 12:

1. Squats: An exercise for conditioning muscles of the legs and buttocks. It can be performed with or without additional weights.

Stand erect with feet about shoulder width apart. Keeping your back straight and head up, slowly bend the knees to squat down, and then return to the standing position. If the knees are bent fully, tremendous mechanical strains are imposed on the joint and can cause irreparable damage. Therefore, the knees are bent only to the half- to two-thirds position. The back is kept straight to reduce the strain on the knees and lower back, and movements should always be slow and controlled.

Squats with additional weights are usually performed with either the barbell resting at the back of the neck (back squat) or across the front of the shoulders and top of the chest (front squat). Both types of squat develop leg, hip, and back strength, but the front squat places more stress on the quadriceps.

There are at least eight other types of squat, each with their own specific advantages and disadvantages. Squats have been called the 'king of all exercises' by some body-builders. If performed properly, squats can greatly strengthen the muscles (especially the quadriceps), bones, tendons, and ligaments in the legs. However, if performed excessively or with poor technique, they can cause a host of stress injuries, including arthritis and torn cartilage of the knee.[8]

2. Dead lifts: A weight-training exercise in which a barbell is picked up from a rack or the floor and slowly brought up to thigh height. It is a simple exercise that increases mobility of the thighs, hips, and lower back muscles, and increases the strength of the back and abdominal areas.

Stand upright, with feet a shoulder's width apart. Bend your legs in order to pick up the barbell and then straighten them to lift it; keep your back and arms straight during the lift; make your legs do most of the hard work.[9]

---

[8] http://www.answers.com/topic/squat
[9] http://www.answers.com/topic/dead-lift

3. Power Cleans and Clean and Jerk:

Power Cleans

A weight-training exercise that develops all-round explosive power by strengthening the legs, trunk, and shoulder girdle muscles. This is an advanced lift and is not recommended for young or novice exercisers. You should always wear a weight belt when performing a power lift.

Crouch down, feet shoulder width apart. Lean forward to grip the bar firmly with an overhand grasp. Before you start the lift, your back and arms should be straight, hips low, shoulders just forward of the bar, and eyes focused forwards. Use your thighs to initiate the lift and then pull power-fully with your upper body to bring the bar to your shoulders in one movement. Keep the bar close to your body. Bend your knees quickly and force your elbows under the bar to 'catch' it. Hop slightly forward between the extension and catch and bend your knees into a slight squat position to receive the barbell at your shoulders. Do not hook the bar over in an arch at the top of the pull. This will cause the bar to hit your chest, pushing it backwards and imposing an unnecessary strain on your lower back. Lower the bar first onto your thighs and then to the floor.[10]

Clean and Jerk

A lift in weightlifting in which a weight is raised from the floor to shoulder height, held there briefly, and then pushed overhead in a rapid motion of the arms, typically accompanied by a spring or lunge from the legs.[11]

4. Bench Press: A relatively simple weight-lifting exercise for toning up arm muscles (particularly the triceps brachii), the anterior deltoids in the shoulder, and the pectorals in the chest. It is usually performed with a barbell.

Lie with your back on a bench and feet flat on the end (or on the floor). Grip the barbell tightly; your palms should face towards your feet, and your arms should be positioned so that you can push vertically upwards. Push slowly against the weights until your arms are fully extended. After holding the extended position, gently lower the weights and return to the starting position. Breathe out when your arms are straightened and in when they are bent. It is important that your lower back maintains contact with the bench.

---

[10] http://www.answers.com/topic/power-clean
[11] http://www.answers.com/topic/clean-and-jerk

The bench press is one of the three lifts in the sport of power lifting and is used extensively in weight training, bodybuilding, and other types of fitness training to develop the chest.[12]

5. Bent-over Rows: This weight-training exercise simulates a rowing action and strengthens the shoulder muscles and biceps in the arm. It can be performed with free weights or at a bench press station on an exercise machine. A bent-over row is a weight training exercise that targets the latissimus dorsi muscle. The bent over row is a much used exercise in training for both bodybuilding and power lifting as it is a good exercise for increasing strength if carried out correctly.

From a standing position, bend down to the floor to hold a barbell with an overhand grasp (palm down). Your hands should be slightly more than shoulder width apart, your upper trunk parallel to the floor, your knees slightly bent, and your feet apart. Keep your trunk parallel to the floor and pull the barbell directly up to your chest, then return to the start position and repeat the movement.[13]

6. Barbell Lunges: A lunge is a position assumed when standing with one leg to the front, knee bent, and the other leg stretched out backwards. When the body is inclined forwards, most of the weight is on the front leg and the muscles of the rear leg are stretched. Lunges are performed as a warm-up exercise for the legs and buttocks.

Stand upright with your feet slightly apart and with your back straight. Take a step forwards with the left leg and bend the knee forwards so that it is directly above the foot. The right leg should be extended backwards with the knee touching (or almost touching) the floor as a result of the movement. The knees should be bent only to a 90° angle. Put your left hand on your left knee and lower your buttocks slightly to increase the stretch in the muscles of the extended leg. Swap legs and repeat.[14]

(In the case of "barbell lunges" you will hold a barbell across your back, resting on your shoulders just as you would during squats and you perform walking lunges carrying the weight).

7. Military "Shoulder" Press: The military press is a variation of the overhead press weight training exercise.

---

[12] http://www.answers.com/topic/bench-press
[13] http://www.answers.com/topic/bent-over-row
[14] http://www.answers.com/topic/lunges

The military press targets the deltoid muscles in the shoulders. Additionally, it works the core and legs, because the lifter must use them to help stabilize the weight. The lift begins with the lifter standing heels together and the barbell on the anterior deltoids. The lifter then raises the barbell overhead by pressing the palms of his hands against the underside of the barbell.

Lift the weighted barbell up to your shoulders, breathing in as you do so. As with all lifts, keep your back straight and use your legs to execute the movement. Hold the barbell on your shoulders for a few seconds and breathe out. Then lift the weights above your head by fully extending your arms. Hold for a few seconds. Gently lower the barbell to your chest then immediately push up again. Repeat the pressing action about four times before slowly lowering the barbell to the ground. Remember to continue breathing throughout the exercise; at no time should you hold your breath.[15]

8. Leg Press: A strength-training exercise done at a leg press station on a weight-training machine. It is popular among sprinters and other runners because it puts little strain on the back. The muscles worked include the quadriceps, gastrocnemius, soleus, and gluteals.

Place your feet flat on the foot rests. Your legs should be bent at 90 degrees at the knee, and your hands should be grasping the seat handles. Fully extend your legs and thighs then return to the start position. Keep your backside on the seat and your back against the backrest throughout the exercise.

Additional Definition: The leg press is a weight training exercise in which the individual pushes a weight away from them using their legs. The term *leg press* also refers to the apparatus used to perform this exercise. The leg press can be used to evaluate an athlete's overall lower body strength (from knee joint to hip and partially ankle extenders as well).

There are two main types of leg press:

- The diagonal or vertical 'sled' type leg press. Cast iron weight disks (plates) are attached directly to the sled, which is mounted on rails. The user sits below the sled and pushes it upward with their feet. These machines normally include adjustable safety brackets that prevent the user from being trapped under the weight.

- The 'cable' type leg press, or 'seated leg press', commonly found on multi-gyms. The user sits upright and pushes forward with their feet

---

[15] http://www.answers.com/topic/military-press-1

onto a plate that is attached to the weight stack by means of a long steel cable.[16]

9. Barbell Shrugs:

Preparation: Stand holding barbell with an overhand or mixed grip; shoulder width or slightly wider.
Execution: Elevate shoulders as high as possible. Lower and repeat.

Since this movement becomes more difficult as full shoulder elevation is achieved, height criteria for shoulder elevation may be needed. For example, raising the shoulders until the slope of the shoulders become horizontal may be considered adequate depending upon individual body structure.[17]

10. Pull-ups: A pull-up is an upper body compound pulling exercise where the body is suspended by extended arms, gripping a fixed bar, then pulled up until the elbows are bent and the head is higher than the hands, utilizing an overhand (pronated) grip. A traditional pull-up relies on upper body strength with no swinging or "kipping" (using a forceful initial movement of the legs in order to gain momentum). The exercise targets mainly the Latissimus Dorsi muscle in the back along with many other assisting muscles.ý Pull-ups are similar to chin-ups, which are distinct due to the underhand (supinated) grip. The difference is that palms are facing away from you in pull-ups, while in chin-ups the palms face yourself. When your arms are not fully extended when doing a pull-up, it is still considered a pull-up.[18]

11. Barbell Bicep Curls: Although the exercises differ, a common factor of each is a 'curling' motion, where a weight—attached to an item of equipment—is moved through an arc, primarily using the strength of the biceps. The biceps is contracted to lift the weight upward through the arc, to a point where further movement is not possible. It is important that the elbow remain next to the body during this motion as to keep stress on the biceps. The biceps is then extended, lowering the weight back through the arc, to the start position. This contraction and extension together constitute a single repetition.

Several variations on the biceps curl transfer some of the load from the biceps to other flexors of the elbow. One group of variations involves postures that hold the elbows in front of the trunk, shortening the biceps and

[16] http://www.answers.com/topic/leg-press
[17] http://www.exrx.net/WeightExercises/TrapeziusUpper/BBShrug.html
[18] http://www.answers.com/topic/pull-up

forcing the brachialis to do more work. Variations on this theme include the preacher curl where the elbows rest upon a sloped bench, the concentration curl where the elbow is braced against the inside of the knee, and the prone incline curl performed lying prone on an inclined bench, where the force of gravity holds the upper arms in front of the trunk.

The biceps curl is usually performed with the palms supinated (facing upwards). Turning the palms inward transfers load from the biceps to the brachioradialis. Variations on this concept include the hammer curl, performed with the palm inward, neither pronated nor supinated, and the reverse curl, with the palms pronated (facing downwards). Another variation, the Morelli Curl uses a traditional over-under or power lifting grip with one palm supinated and the other pronated. The concentric component of the lift is emphasized in the pronated arm, while the eccentric component emphasizes the supinated arm.[19]

12. Weighted Dips: The exercise is done in between parallel bars or facing either direction of trapezoid bars found in some gyms. Feet are crossed with either foot in front and the body is lowered until the elbows are in line with the shoulders. The subject then pushes his/herself up until his/her arms are fully extended, but without locking his/her elbows. This process is then repeated. Dips focus primarily on the chest, triceps, and deltoids.[20] (In the case of "weighted" dips, a belt can be worn with weights attached using a chain, or the weight lifter can grasp a dumbbell between their crossed feet, squeezing it in place using their calves, and perform the dips with additional resistance from added weights).

Honorable Mention Exercises:
- Core exercises for midsection such as hanging leg raises and static holds
- Power lifting techniques such as tire flips and stone lifting
- Heavy machine exercises that focus on pushing or pulling
- Heavy bodyweight exercises
- Lower body exercises involving the largest muscles in the body
- Rowing movements
- Dumbbell exercises
- Any calisthenic exercise with added weights, such as push-ups with a heavy weight on your back

---

[19] http://www.answers.com/topic/biceps-curl
[20] http://www.answers.com/topic/calisthenics

In my bodybuilding program there is still a use for machine exercises, cable exercises, and isolation exercises. I believe compound exercises are most beneficial, but it can still be beneficial to support compound exercises with isolation and machine exercises. These can add much more diversity and fun to your training program when included. I just wouldn't make isolation exercises your priority if adding strength and muscle is your ultimate goal.

The best time to utilize machine and isolation exercises is when warming up prior to starting the free weight workout and after completing all compound free-weight exercises. Using machines before or after your primary workout is a great way to burn out muscles and get them really pumped up. Machines also work well to give your body a break from the intense stress of lifting heavy free weights all the time. Sometimes a day full of machine exercises exclusively is just what the body needs to have joints supported, get deep fluid contractions, and keep good form from start to finish.

Just as there is room for machine and isolation exercises even when choosing the best exercises for the best results in bodybuilding, there is room for other forms of lifting as well. These include power lifting exercises and non-traditional exercises found in manual labor such as lifting and stacking hay bales. Manual labor deserves merit when it comes to building a great physique. From our ancestors to our friends who are farmers or those who lift heavy objects daily in their jobs, many people find ways to stay strong and fit just in day-to-day activities. There is room for all of these training styles in an effective bodybuilding program. Clearly the emphasis should be on compound free-weight exercises; but machines, isolation exercises, and manual labor are all ways to support your bodybuilding goals and contribute to your physique gains. My experience tells me that by incorporating a variety of training methods, a diversity of muscle groups are trained and some muscle groups get a needed break when pounding heavy weights starts to take a toll and wear them down.

Thinking that you can achieve your best physique ever on machines and isolation exercises only is a fantastically erroneous idea. Bodybuilders often marginalize the role of machine exercises. Machines can do a great job but not the best job, and that is where the variety comes in and where special attention to what works best comes into play. It is profoundly unlikely to see top bodybuilders or successful bodybuilders who don't use many of the top 12 muscle-building exercises I suggested; it is as common as long distance running in preparation for a marathon. Lifting heavy free weights impacts the whole body which leads to impressive results. If you do decide to stick to isolation exercises only and have visions of being a top bodybuilder, prepare to be disappointed because results may not come as easily or as quickly as you hope. There is a popular expression for training that says, "Shut up and squat." I can't necessarily pass on that advice as if I follow it because I don't squat due to my back injuries, but I agree with its sentiment. Lifting big will make you big.

My advice would be to—with caution, care, and responsibility—squat, dead lift, press, and pull yourself to a great physique, then eat, rest, recover, and repeat. "Train Hard and Eat Plenty" are words that stretch across a t-shirt my friend Leonard Bakulo from Estonia gave me after we spent six months as training partners back in 2002. I support that concept, and it supports the idea of training to be your best and eating in ways that support your progress and your visions.

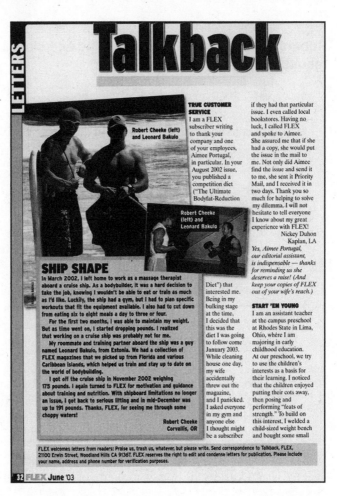

Leonard and Robert featured in a 2003 issue of FLEX Magazine

LETTERS

Talkback

Robert Cheeke (left) and Leonard Bakulo

TRUE CUSTOMER SERVICE

I am a FLEX subscriber writing to thank your company and one of your employees, Aimee Portugal, in particular. In your August 2002 issue, you published a competition diet ("The Ultimate Bodyfat-Reduction Diet") that interested me. Being in my bulking stage at the time, I decided that this was the diet I was going to follow come January 2003. While cleaning house one day, my wife accidentally threw out the magazine, and I panicked. I asked everyone in my gym and anyone else I thought might be a subscriber if they had that particular issue. I even called local bookstores. Having no luck, I called FLEX and spoke to Aimee. She assured me that if she had a copy, she would put the issue in the mail to me. Not only did Aimee find the issue and send it to me, she sent it Priority Mail, and I received it in two days. Thank you so much for helping to solve my dilemma. I will not hesitate to tell everyone I know about my great experience with FLEX!

Nickey Duhon
Kaplan, LA

Yes, Aimee Portugal, our editorial assistant, is indispensable — thanks for reminding us she deserves a raise! (And keep your copies of FLEX out of your wife's reach.)

Robert Cheeke (left) and Leonard Bakulo

SHIP SHAPE

In March 2002, I left home to work as a massage therapist aboard a cruise ship. As a bodybuilder, it was a hard decision to take the job, knowing I wouldn't be able to eat or train as much as I'd like. Luckily, the ship had a gym, but I had to plan specific workouts that fit the equipment available. I also had to cut down from eating six to eight meals a day to three or four.

For the first two months, I was able to maintain my weight. But as time went on, I started dropping pounds. I realized that working on a cruise ship was probably not for me.

My roommate and training partner aboard the ship was a guy named Leonard Bakulo, from Estonia. We had a collection of FLEX magazines that we picked up from Florida and various Caribbean islands, which helped us train and stay up to date on the world of bodybuilding.

I got off the cruise ship in November 2002 weighing 175 pounds. I again turned to FLEX for motivation and guidance about training and nutrition. With shipboard limitations no longer an issue, I got back to serious lifting and in mid-December was up to 191 pounds. Thanks, FLEX, for seeing me through some choppy waters!

Robert Cheeke
Corvallis, OR

START 'EM YOUNG

I am an assistant teacher at the campus preschool at Rhodes State in Lima, Ohio, where I am majoring in early childhood education. At our preschool, we try to use the children's interests as a basis for their learning. I noticed that the children enjoyed putting their cots away, then posing and performing "feats of strength." To build on this interest, I welded a child-sized weight bench and bought some small

FLEX welcomes letters from readers: Praise us, trash us, whatever, but please write. Send correspondence to Talkback, FLEX, 21100 Erwin Street, Woodland Hills CA 91367. FLEX reserves the right to edit and condense letters for publication. Please include your name, address and phone number for verification purposes.

32 **FLEX** June '03

Robert's Recap of choosing the exercises that yield the best results

Seriously consider using the exercises listed above to help you achieve your best results in bodybuilding. If you don't know how to do the exercises correctly, ask an experienced weight lifter at your gym; ask a personal trainer or a bodybuilder and get feedback to make sure you are doing them correctly. Compound exercises are ones you want to do correctly because if you don't, they could lead to injury and setbacks. If there are only a few exercises you choose to do or choose to make time for, squats, dead lifts, and bench press would be the big three I suggest. If you don't have access to a lot of equipment and still want to make the most of your training, choose pull-ups, dips, and explosive power exercises that challenge you to push yourself hard. Be careful; have fun; bring out your best ever physique by incorporating the best possible exercises into your training program.

Robert's Top 10 tips for choosing the exercises that yield the best results

1. Evaluate the exercises that have worked to build muscle for some of the biggest and strongest people throughout history. Use proven techniques to build your physique using the best tools available.

2. If there are power exercises you cannot do because of an injury or muscle weakness in a specific area, determine the best alternative exercises that you can do and apply them to achieve similar results as someone who can do the primary exercises without problems.

3. Learn how to use proper form from experienced weight lifters, and practice your technique to get the most benefit from the exercise and to keep yourself healthy and injury-free.

4. Select a gym that has the appropriate equipment. Some gyms don't allow dead lifts (because they make a lot of noise and can cause injury if done improperly), and if that is an exercise you want to incorporate into your program because of its benefits, then you'll need to factor that into your gym selection.

5. Support your exercise efforts with strong nutrition efforts. It's a shame to put in all the hard work selecting the best exercises if you're not selecting the best food options to help you improve.

6. There are variations for all the best exercises: front squats as opposed to regular squats, decline versus incline bench presses, etc. Use a variety of power movement variations to keep the exercises

exciting and challenging and to target the same muscles in different ways while working additional muscles.

7.　Ask a lot of questions when you see others who have accomplished what you're trying to accomplish; learn from their mistakes and from their success.

8.　Be consistent with your training to allow your body the chance to adapt. When you're doing the best exercises, you'll find that they are exhausting. This is not by accident. In many cases, the harder we work the more we achieve. This isn't always true, but it rings true in the gym regularly. These power exercises will wear you out, but if you get enough rest, enough food, and have enough enthusiasm, you'll keep consistent and see real progress.

9.　Use a spotter to help you move heavy weights. I can't stress this enough. There are so many times I could have prevented injury if only I had someone watching me and helping me get through the movement of the exercise properly. You can't progress if you're taking steps backward because of injury. Use a spotter to keep yourself moving forward.

10.　Make sure that the exercises that yield the best results make up the bulk of your training program. Other exercises have their appropriate place, purpose, and function; but make it a point to spend most of your time doing the exercises that will give you the best results.

"I've known Robert since we were both about crib age. Ever since I can remember, he has had a passion for wrestling. Not the Olympic sport but rather the entertainment sport that many of us associate with Hulk Hogan. It's phenomenal that he has stayed true to his dream of bodybuilding entertainment. Not only has Robert been successful as a bodybuilder, but he has reached this point without putting any toxins in his body—no steroids, no drugs or alcohol, not even any meat or dairy products. He is very influential because he leads by example and doesn't compromise when it comes to what he stands for."

Dylan Kasprzyk
Comedian, Radio Sales Representative, long-time friend
Portland, OR

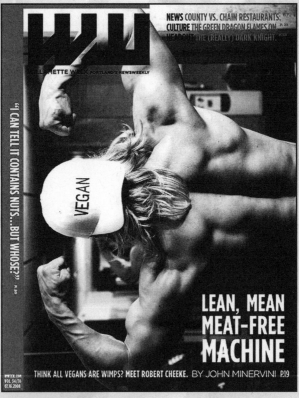

Robert on the cover of the Willamette Week, one of Oregon's most popular newspapers

Chapter 8

Turning your Bodybuilding Success into a Form of Effective Activism and Outreach

"One farmer says to me: 'You cannot live on vegetable foods solely, for it furnishes nothing to make bones with,' walking all the while he talks behind his oxen, who with vegetable-made bones jerk him and his lumbering plow along in spite of every obstacle."

Henry David Thoreau
American author, poet, naturalist

Like many people who follow a vegan lifestyle, I have been involved in protests, boycotts, leafleting, and other forms of direct action activism and outreach promoting veganism and opposing animal cruelty. With more than a decade of experience as an outspoken vegan activist, I can say with confidence and certainty that nothing I have done has been a more effective form of activism than building my body and leading by positive example as a vegan bodybuilder. For me, nothing comes close to the impact I have been able to have on others than the role of vegan bodybuilder. Being something other than what most people expect you to be causes others to take notice; it gets them to pause for a few moments and think differently about veganism.

If you want to have the greatest impact for the vegan movement, it would behoove you to not fit the general stereotype of vegan weakling. I don't oppose that stereotype because I think it is quite true. I believe many vegans do fit into that category of being "vegan weaklings" and that is precisely one of the reasons I work so hard to be anything than what someone would expect when they hear the label "vegan." It is true that most vegans I see appear to be underweight or unhealthy in some way. That just seems to be the way it is. I've traveled all over the country to more vegetarian and vegan festivals than most and observed this reality. Of course it doesn't apply to all vegans, just like any stereotype; but I can fully understand where the stereotype comes from, and it's hard to argue against it without working to change it. Even as a bodybuilder, I still fear that I fit the stereotype when I'm not at my best. It motivates me to work harder to be a better activist and be a better role model for people.

Effective vegan outreach comes down to being a positive and inspirational role model. There are vegan activists who are passionate about saving animal lives and work tirelessly to do so but appear to be unhealthy. This detracts from the message they are trying to promote. So often, passionate activists who really care about animals diminish their efficacy because of the way they look; they turn people away from veganism because the general public associates that image of a skinny, weak, and unhealthy body to animal rights and the vegan lifestyle. Even with good intentions, sometimes vegans cause harm to the animal rights movement when they are not very good physical representatives of the lifestyle. I don't mean to suggest that every vegan must be fit and muscular or meet a certain physical standard, but I'm writing directly about effective activism and what creates positive or negative results as I have perceived it.

If vegans are to be as effective as possible in supporting the vegan movement, they will have to come together as a community to change the image of veganism. Just imagine for a moment if the general, widely accepted image of a vegan was a fit, energetic, positive, caring person who looked healthy and strong and led by positive example by their actions. What could that do for the movement? It could do amazing things and create incredible amounts of change. Right now, vegans are often seen as weaklings, as aggressors, and as those who don't care about health or body image but do care to tell you what you should and shouldn't be doing. I believe vegans can change this image by changing their diets, changing their exercise programs, and ultimately changing their lifestyles. These changes will not only benefit the vegan person's own health and happiness, but also will benefit the vegan movement as they become more effective leaders in their daily lives.

I go out of my way to stand up and represent myself as something different than what people expect. It has led to my most effective activism to date. I'm not even exceptionally muscular and I get people who are amazed, mesmerized, and sometimes stumble over their speech at a loss for words when they see my body and learn that I am vegan. This especially happens at the gym when I am pumped up or when I am wearing my Vegan Bodybuilding & Fitness clothing that is fairly tight fitting and displays what I have worked so hard to achieve physically. This gives people a whole new perspective on veganism. After seeing what I've accomplished as a vegan athlete, many people are inspired to do the very same thing. Even if they don't get excited to pursue veganism, they will likely tell five to ten people about their experience meeting a vegan bodybuilder. The word spreads and gets people thinking differently.

Vegan icon, spokesperson, and influential leader Howard Lyman, Author of *Mad Cowboy* and *No More Bull*, said of me and my lifestyle, "Robert, you're the greatest billboard in the world. People look at you and look up at your hat that displays, 'VEGAN' and say, 'Oh my God, I didn't know they could do that.'" Howard was referring to the fact that as a vegan bodybuilder, I don't look like most vegans or what people expect most vegans to look like, therefore making me an example of what type of physique is possible to attain on a vegan diet. My body, built by a vegan diet, gives hope and inspiration to vegans and non-vegans alike and speaks volumes for the movement, much louder than I could speak using a megaphone on a street corner. My image reaches everyone who sees me in a magazine, on a website, or in a restaurant with far greater dispersion than I could affect with words alone. One of the best parts of being a vegan bodybuilder isn't inspiring vegans to lift weights, eat well, and build their own physiques, but rather seeing the non-vegans who are inspired because they always worried they would get skinny, lose too much muscle, appear weak or less masculine, and never gave veganism a second thought until they saw someone who did it—not just someone who was 200 pounds and maintained it after turning vegan, but someone who was built vegan from childhood. That is a very rewarding feeling and an incredibly effective form of outreach in itself.

When I protest, demonstrate, or leaflet, I may reach dozens or hundreds of people; but when I am featured in mainstream magazines, newspapers, television, and websites as someone who is extremely fit and who lives a vegan lifestyle, I can reach millions. Undoubtedly, there is a need for protests, demonstrations, and more ways to promote veganism through direct activism; but with 1,440 minutes in a day, I want to write books, write magazine articles, and complete interviews for websites to reach millions rather than hundreds and have a greater overall impact. Think for a minute and try to quantify the magnitude of the influence you can have on others in a positive way simply by eating good foods and exercising—basics you should be doing everyday anyway just for overall health—and letting people know about it through your outreach. Imagine what might be if all vegans got on the same page for the common goal of reducing animal suffering by changing the common stereotype associated with the vegan lifestyle and movement.

When you follow a vegan bodybuilding lifestyle and are public about it, you automatically become an activist and role model whether you intend it or not. You demonstrate a reality that most don't think is possible on a pure plant-based diet. I see this happen all the time in my community and on my vegan bodybuilding website. Those who stand out with uniquely strong-looking physiques as vegans become role models instantly and then serve as a resource to which many people direct their friends and family. It illustrates how actions speak louder than words; a muscular or fit physique speaks great volumes to many audiences and has the ability to resonate with people who are working toward accomplishing the same thing in their lives. Being a vegan bodybuilder can make you a more effective activist without the exhaustion of day-to-day battles in arguments, protests, and defense of your lifestyle choices to those who may overlook your message based on your physical appearance. Imagine how effective you could be if you do build your body as a vegan athlete and then go do protests, leafleting, and direct activism. You'd still be doing the type of activism that you enjoy—the face-to-face encounters—but you'll be fit, muscular, and healthy looking and will display a totally different image which completely changes your message. It would give you more credibility. Your image would provide to your audience a different perspective on veganism. Being a vegan bodybuilder basically makes everything you do with activism and outreach more effective. If you took it a step further and decided to use your image and your success story in articles submitted to websites, magazines, and newspapers, you'd reach even more people and further your impact and your outreach efforts.

I'll share some stories from my life to give you some examples of how vegan bodybuilding can be an excellent form of activism and outreach:

When I began this journey of becoming a vegan bodybuilder fifteen years ago, I really didn't know the impact it would have on my life, on the lives of people I would meet, or on the lives of the animals I would save. From the outset, I knew I would make a difference and that I would stand out, but I didn't know how far into mainstream media I would take myself. In the early days back in the mid 1990's, I encouraged other people to adopt a vegan lifestyle through my positive attitude, my successful high school athletic career, and meaningful conversations. I probably only impacted a few dozen people or maybe a hundred during my teenage years. I simply didn't have a big platform for influence other than classes at school and the sports teams I was on. Even then, I got kicked out of class sometimes for my arguments supporting veganism and challenging other ideas. I was a dietary and lifestyle minority on my sports teams. Then the Internet wave came along during my latter years of high school, and I embraced it.

During the rise of the Internet age, I was a young, savvy, ambitious vegan athlete determined to use this medium to reach many more people. I created my own website in 2002 (www.veganbodybuilder.com/

www.veganbodybuilding.com) and have received well over 10,000 e-mails over the years and have reached millions from my presence on over 300 websites making a strong global impact for veganism. I later created many more websites focused around the theme of vegan bodybuilding and fitness. I was one of the early users of myspace.com where I continued my online activism and continued to grow my brand and my name. I spent hours on Myspace to build my personal brand and invited lots of people to become part of my veganbodybuilding.com online forum community. I worked my 7AM to 4PM job and dedicated all other waking hours, aside from gym time, to online social media years before the expression was formed. It worked, and my website grew like crazy as I was able to search keywords and find people around the world who were interested in the same things I was interested in and bring them together to be part of a central community. I made friends, built relationships, inspired many, and grew my website in major ways. For the first time in my life I was able to show the mainstream worldwide audience a side of veganism it had probably never seen before.

With the success my website was experiencing, I decided to start submitting articles and photos to magazines. As a result, I was published and featured in magazines with millions in readership including features in FLEX Magazine for three consecutive years. That is the kind of impact one can have through a vegan bodybuilding lifestyle, and I am honored to be one of the pioneers of this modern era of the industry. It is extremely fulfilling and rewarding for me to share my stories in magazines which makes it exceptionally fun for me to go down this road of activism in the world of mainstream media. And I'm not the only one. My friend and fellow vegan athlete Brendan Brazier has been in far more magazine issues and has written two best-selling books. A co-star in my first documentary along with Brendan, vegan athlete and activist Tonya Kay, is routinely on network television and starred in the 2008 country music video of the year. Vegan bodybuilder Alexander Dargatz has been featured in lots of mainstream media as well, especially in Germany where he lives and has a large following. My very good friend and best-selling author Ani Phyo makes magazine covers and promotes veganism in her print features. She is not only a great role model for our movement but also has been one of my training partners and lives a similar lifestyle of leading by positive example and being fit, healthy, and happy.

Media and technology are the best resources for vegans to advance the cause. Websites, blogs, interviews, and features on television, radio, magazines, and newspapers are incredibly effective outlets. Being up to date with opportunities that are available through media may be the best chance vegans have to reach the most people. As a vegan bodybuilder, you can give the media something interesting and positive to write or talk about. By far the most common online activism today is done through popular social media websites, specifically Facebook and Twitter. MySpace, the first major social media website, paved the way. After Facebook and Twitter— which are used to grow networks and communities, share ideas, news, and status updates—blogs and forums are the next most popular platforms for online activism. Today, one can be an outstanding and highly influential animal rights activist while working in pajamas at home. I know that to be true because I have spent countless hours doing it, and I know from the measurable feedback and impact that it wasn't a waste of time. As much as I love online social networking and promoting veganism from my desk, there are many other ways I promote animal rights outside of the easiest and most effective platform of the Internet.

I spread veganism and promote animal rights through my success as a bodybuilder in many ways. Every time I compete in bodybuilding, it is announced over the microphone that I am vegan. I often wear my Vegan Bodybuilding & Fitness clothing items backstage or in the audience when I'm competing. Regardless of my audience, targeted or mainstream, niche or general, I find a way to positively promote veganism through my success as a vegan bodybuilder. Listed at the end of the chapter are some helpful tips to turn your vegan bodybuilding lifestyle into a positive and effective form of activism and outreach.

When I tour around the country giving talks, I have a variety of outlines and themes that I focus on in my presentations. One of my talk outlines is directly related to activism and, in fact, it is titled, "Nurturing Activism." I use the following outline for various presentations including annual talks at the National Animal Rights Conference (www.arconference.org):

Nurturing Activism
Bringing out the BEST in YOU
A presentation by Robert Cheeke

Tips to bring out the best in you

- Love what you are doing and spend a significant amount of time doing the things you enjoy most.

- Believe in yourself and really mean it.

- Find a support network that understands you and believes in you.

- Learn from those who have achieved what you are trying to achieve.

- Set specific goals outlining what you want to achieve through your outreach and activism.

- Stay positive and support others in the movement.

- Represent veganism in a positive way as part of outreach and grow the movement.

- Make veganism look practical, creative, fun, easy, and accessible to anyone.

- Thrive rather than just get by. Eat for nourishment rather than stimulation.

- Lift others up and support those working toward the same goals.

- Listen to others as a way to offer solutions and learn something new.

- Appreciate those who have paved the way for us to do what we do.

- Respect what you're doing and what you've done; know you're making a difference.

- Apply what you know rather than just talk about it.

- Get adequate rest and take time for yourself. Rejuvenate when stress levels are high.

- When you speak for those who can't be heard, you're standing up for a group worth fighting for, and that in itself has great value.

- Pick your passion. There are many aspects of outreach and activism and so much to cover. Pick the aspects you're most passionate about, and that is where you'll likely have the most significant impact.

- Enjoy life. Be happy that you're making a difference in the world and saving the lives of those you will never meet. Be happy that you're vegan, not sad because you're vegan.

- Strive for wellness and good health so you can effectively carry out your chosen work and impact those you encounter in a positive light.

As you can see, I focus on a lot of positive ways to be an effective activist without having to be involved in confrontational circumstances, though you can still be positive and effective while being involved in conflict or intense conversation. What I aim to communicate to an audience is the concept that whatever we're doing as forms of activism and outreach, they should be constructed with our very best effort and best positive image in mind. I always work to put my best foot forward, my best physique forward, and my best presentation forward because that is in itself effective outreach and an inspiring form of activism.

Achieving success as a vegan bodybuilder and assembling a talk that you can give as you travel for competitions or give at work or in your regional community is a great way to share your message and inspire others all along the way.

When you succeed and make a name for yourself in any industry, especially a niche industry, you can really create your own success. Not only are you succeeding for yourself but also for your cause.

Whether you enjoy direct action activism, protests, debates, or other forms of outreach, know that the most effective way to positively articulate a message is to lead by positive example and to be a happy, healthy, successful person who shines and who thrives.

Turn your vegan bodybuilding success into something even more meaningful. I have been paving the way for the past ten years, and I am excited to see others taking the torch and running with it, creating their own high levels of success in the industry and making themselves exceptional role models, leaders, and activists. Contact me directly, robert@veganbodybuilding.com. I am sincerely excited to help bring out the best in you because it brings out the best in the vegan movement and in the vegan industry. It does the most good that we can for our animal friends who are counting on us every day to stand up and say to animal cruelty, "no more."

You can learn from me or other vegan athletes. Below is a short list which is growing all the time. Some successful vegan bodybuilders who are worth contacting for advice include the following:

Men:
Robert Cheeke
Jimi Sitko
Giacomo Marchese
Steve Arntt
Joel Kirkilis
Alexander Dargatz
Robbie Hazeley
Kurt Sollanek
Justin Karstetter
Torre Washington
Patrick Reiners
Florian Boge
Manny Escalante
Ed Bauer

Women:
Denise Nicole
Heather Morgan
Kailla Edger
Melissa Brey
Marzia Prince

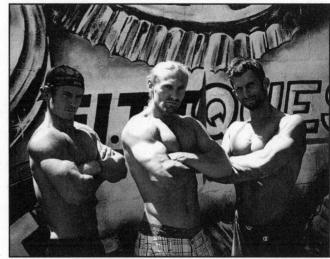

*Vegan Brothers in
Iron: Jimi Sitko,
Robert,
Giacomo Marchese
(photo by
Brian Van Peski)*

All of these individuals can be found on www.veganbodybuilding.com and are part of the website's online forum community. There are many more too. As I referenced earlier, there are nearly 4,000 members on our website so there are a lot of people to network with, connect with, and learn from. The athletes listed above are purely competitive bodybuilders, fitness and figure competitors. There are thousands more involved in other sports, including power lifting and endurance sports. Explore the website and connect with those who's bios and images inspire you the most. We have dozens of featured vegan athletes on our website with proper interviews and bios from endurance athletes like Brendan Brazier, power lifters like Ryan Wilson and Crystal Hammer, fitness models like Koya Webb, and recreational athletes like Julia Abbott.

Get in touch with those who have done what you're trying to do and who have been effective, influential positive role models for many people all over the world.

There are many other vegan athletes in a variety of other sports such as weight lifting and cycling. If your interests in vegan bodybuilding and fitness extend to those sports, please visit the following websites to connect with many of those vegan athletes:

www.veganfitness.net
– An online community forum of vegan athletes

www.organicathlete.org
– A non-profit organization of athletes promoting organic foods

www.veganbodybuilding.org
– A UK-based vegan bodybuilding informational website

www.veganbodybuilding.com
– A website and forum with the theme "Healthy Food Defines You"

Joni Purmonen (veganfitness.net), Bradley Saul (organicathlete.org), and Pete Ryan (www.veganbodybuilding.org) are the leaders of the websites listed in addition to mine. They are all outstanding leaders in the vegan movement and people I consider friends.

If you want to lead by example, the best way is to simply do something that inspires others. The best way to do that authentically is to be true to yourself and do things you're naturally passionate about. Build your physique into something that inspires people. Let people know how you did it. Start writing about it and making yourself visible.

Robert's Recap of ways to turn your bodybuilding success into a form of effective Activism and Outreach

I learned a long time ago that the best way to influence someone to understand your way of thinking is to lead by positive example. I see veganism as a positive thing, and if we go about our lives caring for others and keeping the bigger picture in mind, we should naturally be effective in our activism and outreach. There are specific methods of enhancing our effectiveness as activists, such as living a healthy lifestyle, having a positive attitude, being good listeners, and maintaining a fit and muscular physique that many will be impressed by and associate with veganism. Be confident and outgoing in your communication with others rather than hiding or shying away from positive and influential messages you have to share. Work really hard to do meaningful things you really care about and you will be an effective activist as a result.

Robert's Top 10 tips for turning your bodybuilding success into effective forms of Activism and Outreach

1. Make it known that you are a vegan bodybuilder. Talk with others about your lifestyle and be a role model. Talk about it among your friends. Encourage your vegan friends to build their physiques as well to represent a strong and healthy side of veganism to all those you encounter. The more successful you are as a vegan bodybuilder,

the more effective you can be as an activist, but it doesn't work unless people know about it. Make it a point to let people around you know that you lead a vegan lifestyle, and let your actions speak for themselves.

2. Wear clothing that says "VEGAN" on it. There are countless places to find these clothing items all over the Internet. www.veganbodybuilding.com is a great place to start because the clothing says "Vegan Bodybuilding & Fitness" right on it. Other general websites for vegan clothing are www.veganessentials.com and www.herbivoreclothing.com. There are many other places for awesome vegan clothing all over the Internet too, so search around to find what style fits you. When you wear around clothing that says "VEGAN" on it and you have an athletic physique, your actions speak for themselves and you don't even have to say anything to be an effective activist. People just look at you, read your clothing, absorb the messages, and make the connection. Then, if they are driven to do so, they may approach you and ask you about your lifestyle. This happens to me all the time as a vegan bodybuilder, and it is one of the most effective ways I promote the lifestyle. Get your vegan gear and wear it around!

3. Write articles to vegan and non-vegan publications to share your vegan bodybuilding lifestyle publicly.

4. Build your own website; start your own blog; film your own videos about your success as a vegan athlete. There is a huge audience for this, and it is a fantastic form of activism and outreach, especially showcasing your unique lifestyle.

5. When you succeed in a competition and are proud of your results, tell a local newspaper or even a national newspaper or magazine and share your story with them. Anyone can compete in bodybuilding, vegan or non-vegan. Anyone can win in bodybuilding, vegan or non-vegan. But one is far more interesting to publications and audiences and that of course is the combination of vegan and bodybuilding. Tell your story and get some media press around it which then reaches masses of people rather than a small regional audience of friends, family, and acquaintances.

6. Have meaningful conversations with other people and express yourself honestly, telling them the story of your own journey to becoming a vegan bodybuilder.

7. Enjoy what you are doing and allow your enthusiasm to be evident among those around you. Inspire others through the pure enjoyment of your lifestyle. Be a friendly, outgoing, and positive spokesperson for the vegan and animal rights movements. The best way to create change is from leading by positive example.

8. Network with vegan groups and organizations and offer to give presentations to their members or write for their newsletters. Partner with non-profit animal rights organizations to help them reach different audiences. Offer to be a spokesperson for them, volunteer for them, and help bring more attention to their organization through your own outreach. They will also be able to promote you and you can work harmoniously together towards a common goal.

9. Work hard to get yourself sponsored by companies or organizations which will give you more exposure and a greater platform to effectively represent your lifestyle.

10. Learn from other vegan bodybuilders—from their mistakes and from their successes. Many methods for effective activism have been tried. Find out what works.

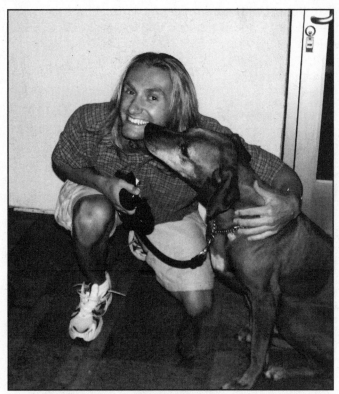

Robert with Ani Phyo's companion friend Kanga

"I have known Robert since before he was a 98-lb weakling. As a friend of his since middle school, I have seen Robert tackle many challenges. He strives for excellence and success in whatever he does. He started one of the top vegan websites without knowing HTML, became a top sales person without having a sales background, and became a champion bodybuilder after being a skinny kid. Next, Robert will be a successful writer. There is no one more qualified to write about being a vegan and successful athlete. Robert lives it every day."

Nick Martin
Software developer, Entrepreneur, Author
Corvallis, OR

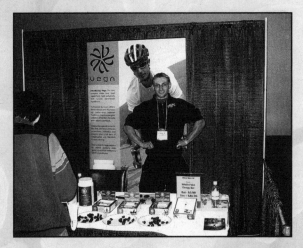

Working for Vega for the first time in 2005 in Vancouver, BC

Photo of Robert on the front door at the HELD Vegan Belt Store in Portland, OR

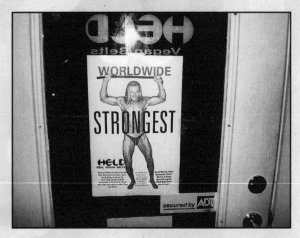

Chapter 9

How to Market Yourself to get Sponsored

"I see incredible opportunities lost every day because people with seemingly unlimited potential don't know how to effectively turn it into something productive. This saddens me but also inspires me to reach out and help them achieve."

Robert Cheeke, Author

Getting sponsored by a company is one of the primary goals all bodybuilders have. When we finally do get sponsored it is an incredibly exciting time, equivalent to winning an award for a meaningful achievement. It's the realization that the hard work has paid off and finally it's time for recognition and reward. It is truly a destination that we seek and a situation we thrive in once achieved. It boosts self esteem, gives us something to take great pride in, and helps us find more meaning in our sport. No matter what our interests are, there are companies out there who share the same interests and would likely consider working with us and collaborating with us to spread a message that both parties share a common interest in.

I've been around the bodybuilding industry for a full decade and I am constantly amazed by some of the top bodybuilders in the world who seemingly have no clue how to market themselves in any measurable way. Some of the best bodybuilders in the world currently don't have major sponsors, aren't being used in advertising, and are getting little to no publicity because they don't know how to effectively market and present themselves. They have outstanding physiques they worked hard for, but nobody is even paying attention. In the marketing and personal fulfillment aspects of bodybuilding, that is a travesty. Sure, they are bodybuilders, not sales people or marketing gurus, but they should know how to present themselves better than they seem to be doing to have a more rewarding and influential career. The bridge between bodybuilder and marketer needs to be formed, and that gap between athlete and representation of a company needs to be narrowed. In many professional sports, athletes have agents who help them with this aspect of their career. Not many pro bodybuilders I know have agents and most go at it on their own or have their husbands, wives, or partners handle this aspect for them even though it is something they too know little about.

Personal marketing is a fascinating topic to me because I come from a background of making a lot based on a little; turning something small into something big, regardless of what my resources are. I come from a background in bodybuilding but currently have a job in sales. I have paired the two together quite nicely. In fact, I have done so in ways from which I have benefited greatly and have helped others out along the way with my experiences and my success. I come from a background of success in self-marketing and self-promoting, creating opportunities for myself in order to contribute to a greater good and various causes, while I watch those who have so much more potential, much better physiques, and a much more accomplished bodybuilding résumé getting so little exposure and minimizing their careers as a result.

Marketing yourself doesn't have to be hard. In fact, it should be very easy and a lot of fun. Marketing yourself is basically promoting and highlighting your strengths, unique characteristics, talents, and abilities that stand out among a crowd. Attitude plays a major factor in the way that you market yourself and that is the first thing I notice when I evaluate the character of other bodybuilders. The ability to be innovative and creative is extremely important as well and cannot be overlooked. I have had the chance to represent companies such as Bodybuilding.com, the largest bodybuilding company in the world; Sequel Naturals, the 8th fastest growing company in Canada in the Profit 100 rankings in 2008; as well as smaller companies and organizations such as Organic Athlete, Vegan Bodybuilding & Fitness, HELD Vegan Belts, New Grip non-leather weight lifting gloves, VegSeattle, and other products, companies, and organizations. The more experiences I have, the more I learn, and the lessons I learn are things that I can pass along to others to save everyone some time. It also allows me to shed light on the actions I took to secure a position working for some fantastic products, companies, organizations, and people over the years within a variety of industries, including bodybuilding.

Common marketing and self-promotion mistakes made by bodybuilders (even the pros):

If you have ever been to a major bodybuilding competition like the Arnold Schwarzenegger Classic or the Olympia, you have seen massive bodybuilders behind a 10 by 10 foot or larger booth often sitting (not standing) waiting for fans to come by and buy one of their portrait photos of them flexing for $10 each. Many times the expressions on their faces and their body language display to an audience that they are not very approachable and would much rather be somewhere else than at an expo filled with their fans and potential fans. That is about the extent of the average professional bodybuilder's efforts in the form of marking and advertising themselves at a major event. It's a start but it's not getting them very far. I applaud those bodybuilders who do stand behind the booth or even come out in front of it, rather than sitting down being less approachable; and I applaud those who have thought of other things to sell or promote such as their own clothing line, a training DVD, or a book. That takes more thought and more effort than "just" selling $10 photos of yourself as your sole form of marketing. I understand that it is hard to stand for prolonged periods when you are on a low carbohydrate diet before a competition, and I've even thought that it is unfair for the bodybuilding federations and supplement companies to require that the bodybuilders attend the expo the day before their competition, but part of being a pro bodybuilder is interacting with fans, which helps keep the sport alive and going. The better a bodybuilder can interact with the fans and offer them something of value or interest other than a photo of themselves, the better for everyone. I applaud louder for those who are friendly, outgoing, engaging, enthusiastic, and have found their own unique niche within the industry. By far, my favorite all-time bodybuilders are the ones I had pleasant experiences with when meeting them for the first time as a young person and a huge fan of bodybuilding. I will always remember those individuals, and that is how I present myself when meeting my fans as well. I engage and interact with fans sincerely and authentically because of how important my role model's interaction with me was many years ago and the lasting impression it had on me. It actually pains me to some degree to see those with so much potential wasting their abilities by not applying themselves appropriately in terms of building their personal brand, representing the sport of bodybuilding and the companies they endorse, and interacting with the fans in a positive way which keeps the sport alive and growing.

The bodybuilding industry is full of copycats. Not many bodybuilders seem to be doing anything new or unique to further their success. When someone does something outside of the norm it stands out dramatically because everyone else is just copying others. However, it is a system that only works for some, not all. Bodybuilders who are less popular or less photogenic or who are naturally more shy or less friendly are going to have a much harder time selling their photos than someone who is popular, photogenic, and friendly. That's just the way it is. It is time bodybuilders wake up to innovation and start using their imaginations because relying on stagnant techniques in a broken system of attempted self-marketing isn't going to get them anywhere. There is unlimited potential waiting for those who think outside the box of current trends. Find what is popular, what works, and improve on it. As a kid I learned a slogan from my involvement in 4-H, which stated the motto, "Make the Best Better" and that applies directly to bodybuilding and marketing yourself in innovative ways to get sponsored.

If you want to stand out and get noticed so you can get sponsored, which is one of the ultimate goals for bodybuilders (because it helps you get more recognition, helps you financially, gives you more leverage and credibility with your career, etc.), you have to find your own unique advantages and demonstrate them. What makes you more marketable than someone else? What is truly more unique about you? What would make companies want to have you represent them? What can you offer them and what can you do for them and what can you bring to their team? Those questions won't always lead to the same answers. They will reveal your diversity. For example, what makes me marketable? My pleasing-looking physique, my all-American blond hair and approachable, friendly appearance. Additionally, but just as important, my name and reputation make me very marketable. What makes me unique? My vegan diet, vegan bodybuilding lifestyle, and my do-it-myself attitude make me very unique and stand out as one-of-a-kind. What would make companies want me to represent them? My celebrity status and the role-model influence I have on so many people within many different industries would have many companies excited about the opportunity to have me represent them, which is what I've experienced for years. I also have a work ethic that is a standard above what most set for themselves and that is incredibly desirable for any company or organization. What can I offer the company and what can I bring to the team? I can bring years of experience in successful marketing and promotion, a positive attitude, and a history of innovation, creativity, and success to the team. I can also bring a social media network of thousands of people I am connected with via popular social media websites. That alone, is very valuable to a company. Often times you'll be asked, "How big is your network?" or, "How big is your mailing list?" Those statistics reveal a lot about the number of people you are connected with and the type of influence that you have. Overall, I bring my personal brand to the team and with that comes a large network, connections, reputation, and a history of success achieved.

As you can see, each of these primary questions can provide a completely different answer than the others, but they are all related to marking and promoting yourself in ways that can benefit your career and benefit the causes that are meaningful to you. Know who you are, what your talents are, strengths and abilities are, and use those to get what you have worked so hard to earn— sponsorship to help sustain your lifestyle and stimulate your career. Be aware of your weaknesses too and work hard to turn them into strengths.

Once you know who you are and what you want to achieve, how do you discover what sets you apart from the rest? You already figured out what makes you unique and marketable. You have concluded why companies would want to work with you, so now how do you go about making it happen? It begins by taking notice of what is already out there, what is popular, what trends are common throughout the industry and seeing if you fit into those categories. If so, you can proceed following a specific pattern, but if not, you'll need to create your own path and make opportunities for yourself rather than wait for them. It's not all about recognizing your strengths and unique talents but about taking action to use them and do something worthwhile that will get you closer to where you want to be.

By far, the biggest flaw I see in the approach most bodybuilders take is that they lack action to support their goals. Without taking action it is hard to achieve desired results. You can be the most promising, up and coming star, the most talented bodybuilder or fitness model, but if you don't apply yourself, you won't end up getting anywhere. When I observe pro bodybuilders as I travel around the bodybuilding show circuit, I see a lot of things not working for them. I see the same old things from city to city, show to show with no improvement from one year to the next as far as their marketing or their market value goes. I see a lack of creativity and innovation, a shortage of application and effort, cases of apathy, and an attitude that doesn't get them to the next level. Sometimes they get so caught up in themselves they forget why they got into the sport and what their ultimate goals are. Instead, they focus on short-term self-centered agendas. If your effort is minimal, you can expect your results to reflect that.

When I see new creative ways of marketing an athlete in bodybuilding, I get excited because it opens up opportunities, new perspectives, and new approaches that others can model. Some past bodybuilding innovations and approaches have included the production of training videos, clothing lines, personal brand building within social media platforms, and linking up with the mixed martial arts industry, pro wrestling industry, modeling industry and the movie/entertainment industry. Some bodybuilders use a particular physical feature to trademark themselves and build recognition such as a unique facial feature, muscle group that stands out, or tattoo. This is all part of building one's own unique personal brand. Based on my observations, the pro body-builder who has moved forward with the most innovative ideas and who created a demand for his brand by creating his own market is Jay Cutler. He also happens to be the current Mr. Olympia as of 2009, meaning he is the best bodybuilder in the world and is the face and name of bodybuilding today. But even before he was number one, he was building his brand by publishing his own book, creating a new DVD video every year, giving talks all over the country, creating a clothing line, posting weekly videos on his website mak-ing himself accessible to fans, co-branding himself with major supplement companies and stores, and being a friendly, approachable role model for body-building fans all over the world. I respect Jay for always being a step ahead of everyone else and for creating new opportunities rather than waiting for them. I met Jay in 2001, and we became friends over the years and remain friends today. I was the first person to congratulate him in Las Vegas when he won the Olympia for the third time earlier this year. He inspires me greatly because of everything positive that he represents. Read more about Jay on www.jaycutler.com.

I'll share some examples I used for effective marketing of myself as a vegan bodybuilder to earn the opportunities I have had to represent compa-nies, products, and a variety of industries. These approaches also led to enhanced media exposure, a larger social media network, and additional op-portunities that were very fulfilling for me individually and which ultimately furthered my career. Use some of these approaches as models to help you get sponsored, and as always, think of your own unique ideas to make the best better and create your own ideal opportunities.

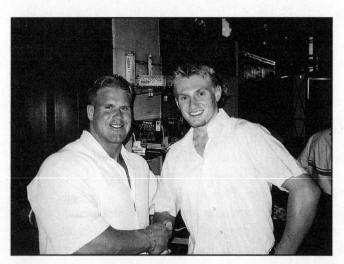

Robert with Mr. Olympia Jay Cutler back in 2001 at the USA Bodybuilding Championships

Promoting yourself to accomplish what you want:

One of the first things I did was create my website www.veganbodybuilding.com. The website enabled me to get international recognition—recognition outside my home town and current community. The website laid the foundation for my ability to network with others and be discovered by people looking for information around the topics I presented and represented.

I gave myself a title early on in my career, just after launching my website, referring to myself as "The World's Most Recognized Vegan Bodybuilder" and then living in ways that reflected that title and making it overwhelmingly true. Giving myself a title, especially such a big and profound title, gave me a high standard to work toward every day, constantly making myself better and reinforcing the validity of that title year after year. The title I gave myself brought more attention to me and the causes I represented, created more opportunities for me to be used in media, and helped me get featured in magazines, newspapers, websites, and on TV and radio shows.

Additionally, I networked with other vegan individuals, business owners, organizations, and groups which added more familiarity and notoriety to my name and gave me an opportunity to have a mutually beneficial relationship with a lot of people around the world. I wrote articles and submitted them to magazines for publicity and to build my résumé, making it much stronger which proved to be an essential aspect of my marketing years down the road.

I had photos taken of me when I was in my best shape. For branding purposes I used the same "best" photos of me over and over in each publication and with each article so that when someone saw that image they knew it was Robert Cheeke, the World's Most Recognized Vegan Bodybuilder.

I worked hard and did all the little things I needed to do that I knew others wouldn't be willing to do. Not many people are willing to work more than 12 hours a day every day. I knew if I did that, I could accomplish more and I would stand out, and that is exactly what happened. I simply worked harder than others and earned the title I still use a decade later. It was a true and fitting title from the onset, but it always motivated me to stay a step ahead of everyone else in fear of losing the title because it meant a lot to me. That simple action ultimately led to a lot of success I likely wouldn't have experienced without a title to live up to everyday.

After I built my foundation I approached others, presented a mutually beneficial proposal to them, and collaborated effectively to further our careers doing things we love to do. I looked for opportunities and I created opportunities rather than waited. I continue to be innovative and every year I produce something that has never been done before. My career has become very sustainable. I was never "here today, gone tomorrow" but have been constantly evolving and improving and building my reputation and market value. I work extremely hard to maintain my good image and integrity and to represent the industries and companies in the most positive ways I can. The primary reason I will never be here today and gone tomorrow is because I never relied too heavily on anyone else but I put in the work from the ground up, day in and day out, and built my own reputation and have a support base that has grown with me and won't be washed away if I leave a certain company or product that I represent. It is fundamentally important to understand this, because if you ever rely on any company too much, everything could be gone tomorrow and you'll have nothing to fall back on. You always need something to fall back on and there is no stronger base than a foundation that you built yourself from the ground up.

Sending Proposals out to get sponsored:

In my early days of bodybuilding I enthusiastically sent proposals out to a variety of companies seeking sponsorship, hoping to represent them. I worked very hard on these efforts back in 2002-2004 but ultimately, nothing came from it. I had my sister and my father help me with some aspects of this because they are much smarter than I and could proof read my material before sending it out. I was determined and focused and went after it with the same passion I have for everything else I wanted to achieve. But in this case, it just didn't work out the way I had planned. There were a variety of reasons why the proposals didn't work out and nearly all of them were directly my fault. Later I would recognize some of the flaws in my attempts and efforts to get sponsored by reaching out to companies I was interested in. One of my biggest mistakes was lack of follow through and being intimidated to call on the phone and speak with the people I needed to. I did make phone calls, in fact quite a few of them, but there were some chances I had to follow through that I just didn't take. I also contacted a lot of the wrong companies. I targeted vegan food companies rather than supplement and performance-enhancing product companies. There were some protein powder companies I contacted. Those were the ones that expressed interest, but I became intimidated as things progressed and didn't follow through properly and ultimately accepted rejection, lost interest, and moved on. I learned a lot of lessons that helped me later on. For example, I recently landed multiple opportunities to work with the largest bodybuilding company in the world, Bodybuilding.com. With Bodybuilding.com I used the power of my social network and the power of my influence on social networks to prove to them that I would be a person who could benefit their company.

When you plan on sending out proposals to product companies, here are some things to keep in mind: Create a list of the companies and products you are interested in and appreciate the most. Make sure the list is sincere because it will enhance and improve your chances of representing a company when you are a true fan of their products. If you struggle with brainstorming this list, simply look around your kitchen at the nutrition products you current pay to use. That should give you an idea of the products you sincerely use and care about. Evaluate the companies to determine which ones are the most reasonable and most likely to have sponsorship opportunities available. Find out which ones you honestly feel you have the best shot at and prioritize them. Some research will need to be done because it will save time, money, and energy in the long run. For example, some companies don't sponsor athletes because they don't have a budget to do so or because it is just part of their company policy or because they have no interest in doing so. Look at the products you have, use, and love and check out the company website, send them an e-mail, or give them a call to find out if they do indeed sponsor athletes and what the procedure is to join their team. Some will be very obvious because you may even see athletes featured on the packaging, in their literature, in advertising, or on their website. Once you've done the research to find out if the companies you like sponsor athletes, inquire about applying to be a sponsored athlete.

It is always a safe option to follow the instructions the website provides and is appropriate to follow-up with an e-mail within a week or two after you've submitted your application.

When you're preparing yourself to contact potential sponsors, it is important to know and understand your résumé and personal brand. If you have been featured in newspapers, in magazines, on websites, or in other forms of media, it is important to have detailed records of those appearances and features organized and ready to be used. It displays a level of commitment, organization, and desire to your potential sponsors. It also sheds light on your accomplishments and your ability to succeed in areas of personal interest. Having that organized collection makes you much more marketable, shows your preparation, and deepens your interest in the eyes of the companies you're seeking. Having these resources available is extremely important, so keep detailed records of all of your awards, media features, and accomplishments. They will come in handy later on down the line. I know this from first-hand experience and it has literally "sealed the deal" for me when I've been able to display to a potential sponsor all the work that I have done in mainstream media and all the recognition I have received, which raises my market value. I even used this approach to secure a literary agent, which I did last year by sending copies of a large assortment of my media exposure from print media and online website features and videos along with my book manuscript to my potential agent, who ultimately signed a contract with me.

If the companies you are seeking sponsorship from do not have online forms to fill out on their website, they will likely have a phone number you can call with inquires or an address to which you can ship a proposal. Again, when preparing a proposal, express your great interest in the company and be as sincere as you can, giving some examples or testimonials from your experiences with their products. Make comments about specific attributes of the company or products that you really like the most and explain to them with confidence how you can bring more attention to their products and bring more business to their company with your sheer enthusiasm for their brand. Provide specific examples to show them exactly how they will benefit from working with you and explain your desire to work for them because of your appreciation and love for their products. Show them the size of your social media networks, examples of the influence you have on others, and your traveling schedule if you're on tour; explain the connections that you have to influential people in various industries.

I know from experience that many companies are looking for genuine fans of their products to represent them and promote them, not just celebrities. Companies will care much more about the people who are already enthusiastic about their products than those they have to try to teach to be enthusiastic about them. Those who naturally love the products are always going to be the best ambassadors even if they aren't as well known or famous. Of course, this isn't always true. Someone like Michael Jordan could sell literally anything because of his name recognition and popularity based on his accomplishments in his sport. But the general rule is the more authentic and sincere you are the better chances you have at being sponsored, which is why finding a harmonious relationship between you and a company you really like is an important aspect in the process of earning sponsorship. Sincere testimonials of product use and success are one of the most common ways to get the attention of any company.

Fill out the necessary sponsor application forms online for submission or send a physical proposal complete with samples of your exposure in media. When you're all ready to send your proposal out, inquire about the name and specific job title of the person you are submitting it to and put that information in the appropriate heading for your proposal. Use standard sizes and fonts and print on good quality plain white paper (use high quality printer paper, not 'photocopy' paper which is lower in weight, not as firm or bright, and not as high quality). Use a standard template with a proper heading, bullet points, clear, crisp, and concise paragraphs with appropriate titles and a summary at the end highlighting the most important points.

In your proposal, include all the appropriate details and information you wish to provide and attach your résumé which should be updated and targeted towards this specific prospect. Once you've created your proposal seeking sponsorship, have others proof-read it for you to get other perspectives and feedback. Make sure it is well constructed, well-written, and very professional. Sign it with blue ink to show it is authentic and original and not a photocopy. Bind it together in whatever format is preferred, usually a simple staple, paper clip, or plastic-bound covering with full-length, left side binding. When totally completed, ship it using a professional folder or document mailer and send it priority mail rather than a standard, parcel post, or slow rate of delivery. Use FedEx, UPS, DHL, or USPS Priority to ensure it gets there quickly and professionally. Follow up after a week or two to see if it has been received and try to set up a time to speak with them to talk about the possibilities of a mutually beneficial working relationship. Be advised that most communication will likely be via e-mail because it is less confrontational than other forms and is very convenient. Don't get discouraged if you're not selected right away or if you don't hear back right away. Often times companies get lots of inquires and it may take them a while to get back to you. While you're waiting to hear back, send proposals to other companies on your list. The process is essentially like looking for a job of any kind, which in essence is what you're doing. You'll have to approach sponsorship like a job search. Being persistent, contacting lots of companies, following up, and keeping a positive outlook and open mind are all parts of this process. In the end, your hard work and persistence will pay off.

Anticipate the questions that you will be asked so when you do get contacted you're ready with answers. This may be related to your ability to travel, potential photo shoot dates (which may mean you'll need to be in shape like the photos you submitted to them displayed), your expectations for compensation, and general expectations that *you* have in the business relationship.

Once you become a sponsored athlete, it is important to represent the company in the ways that you said you would and in the ways that will ensure you'll enjoy the experience and that your employer will want to keep you around. It is important to be mindful, tactful, respectful, punctual, responsible, and very professional, representing the company in a positive way that makes both of you look good. You will always want to be on good terms with your sponsor keeping doors open for additional and future opportunities with them or elsewhere. People within the same industry talk to one another so if you have a bad reputation, word will travel and it will be harder for you to find future sponsors. Look for ways you can go above and beyond expectations as you represent companies. You'll often be rewarded with opportunities you didn't previously have. If you act and behave in the ways you'd like employees behaving for you, you'll be just fine and will do well representing a company you truly care about.

How I got sponsored

When I reflect back on some of my early attempts to get sponsored, I recognize some flaws that I had in my approach. I didn't target my efforts appropriately and failure was my ultimate outcome.

In 2005, I took an innovative approach and did indeed get sponsored. I directed, produced, and starred in my own documentary which gave me exposure and featured a product developer, Professional Ironman Triathlete Brendan Brazier. I didn't recruit Brendan because of his relationship with Vega, the product line he formulates. In fact, at the time I didn't know anything about Vega or Sequel Naturals, the parent company. I just knew that Brendan was a professional vegan athlete and someone I wanted in my documentary. I learned about Vega from Brendan during the filming of our documentary but never imagined I would be working with Vega months later. Just before my documentary was completed I got a surprise phone call from Charles Chang, the President of Sequel Naturals, which produces Vega. Charles asked the questions I referenced earlier. He asked about the size of my network, how many Vegan Bodybuilding & Fitness shirts I sell per month, etc. He asked if I would like to send out a sample packet of Vega along with a brochure to every customer who buys a t-shirt or clothing item from me and if I would be interested in doing the same when the documentary came out in the very near future. I told him I would be delighted to do so, and sure enough, products and literature were sent to my house. He also offered me a sponsorship in exchange, offering me all the free products I wanted because he understood how influential I was in my industry of Vegan Bodybuilding & Fitness. In exchange he used my image and a quote from me about Vega in their updated brochure for the Vega products. Four years later, I remain in the brochure today along with many well known ambassadors and sponsored athletes.

Charles recognized my ability to influence a lot of people, and those people happened to be the same crowd of people he was looking to reach with his products. I later accepted a full-time job with Sequel Naturals in 2006, became the number one salesperson in the country two years later and have been highly influential for their company ever since. In this case, I didn't rely on a proposal inquiring about sponsorship but I allowed my actions, my enthusiasm, and my personal brand to secure the position for me.

I first caught the attention of Vega because I was a person who fit their brand, was a fan and friend of Brendan, and because I had a large community that I have the ability to influence. My job within Sequel Naturals changes dramatically from one year to the next because of the innovation I keep bringing to the table and because of the trust Charles has in me to deliver what I say I will deliver. It was because I was innovative, marketable, and influential that I was able to get the opportunity and thrive. Sequel Naturals features me on their website and brochures and supports my athletic efforts, my personal interests, and my career interests. This builds the "Robert Cheeke" brand along with the Vega brand and both Charles and I see the value in helping our brands grow together. Because I am so marketable, I get offers from various other companies who are interested in sponsoring me. I turn them all down except the ones that don't compete with Vega products because my relationship with Sequel Naturals, Charles Chang, Brendan Brazier, and the whole Vega product line has been so strong for half a decade. Loyalty is a powerful expression of gratitude for opportunities granted and something that should be communicated regularly to your sponsors.

In late July 2009 I created an opportunity to work with Bodybuilding.com for the first time. I contacted them on my own, with Charles' support, asking them to carry the Sequel Naturals product lines on their website. Again, I relied on my personal brand, my social network, and my influence to get the deal worked out and make Sequel Naturals products available on their website. In this case, I did send a proposal with figures, projections, and a long list of ways I would support them. Their website gets over 200,000 unique visitors per day, and I got them to feature Vega on the front of their website. I sent out newsletters to my social networks encouraging people to support Bodybuilding.com and buy Vega products from their website. I even had incentives such as free Bodybuilding.com t-shirts to send out to those who supported Vega, ordering it from their website. I sent the Bodybuilding.com staff samples of our products and other promotional items. I also expressed my sincere appreciation of their company and even mentioned names of their famous spokesmodels that I am friends with or fans of. To further my own personal brand as well as increase sales for Vega on their website, I sent another proposal inviting myself to work at major events representing

Bodybuilding.com and promoting Vega. I never waited to be asked for the opportunity but proactively asked to be involved and was invited to do so.

Sure enough, my personal brand and enthusiasm were appreciated and I worked directly with Bodybuilding.com, at their booth at the 2009 NPC USA Bodybuilding Championships (the event where Mr. America is determined). I was the only non-IFBB Professional bodybuilder or fitness model working the Bodybuilding.com booth, and it was the largest booth at this entire event. I worked hard, displaying my unique character and enthusiasm to the fullest. Days later I received a phone call from the event coordinator for the $200 million company Bodybuilding.com saying, "Robert, you have what just can't be taught. You have the ability to interact with an audience that you just can't teach someone. We have models knocking down our door asking to work for us at the Olympia coming up in September, but you're the first person I'm calling because you have what it takes to stand out and make an impact with us." I was elated, honored, and was pumping my fist with excitement. There are nearly five million people who want the opportunity to work for Bodybuilding.com and especially at the Olympia, the event Arnold Schwarzenegger won seven times for the most prestigious title in bodybuilding.

Millions want the opportunity, and Bodybuilding.com called me first because they observed the abilities that I demonstrated at their booth from the years of experience I have running booths for Sequel Naturals all over the United States. Because I have a good understanding of psychology and communication, I excelled working with Bodybuilding.com at the USA Championships. I did the same in Las Vegas at the Olympia working alongside legends in bodybuilding and role models I've had for ten years. Again, I stood out and took control running the operations at our 80 by 10 foot booth. Managers at Bodybuilding.com praised my efforts and it has led to further opportunities, a strong relationship with Bodybuilding.com, and increased sales of Vega products on their website. This illustrates the win-win situation you are looking for.

In my early days I was young and had accomplished less so I had to do all the groundwork to try to get attention from companies. Over time I realized that if I dedicate more time to improving as an athlete and building up my reputation I would have people coming to me, which is what happens now on a fairly regular basis. You get to this point by working hard and getting lots of media exposure for being unique, innovative, or creative. Vegan Bodybuilding & Fitness is a very unique concept, and since I am the founder of the company and the face of the lifestyle, I get a lot of opportunities. My best advice is to put in the time to create a name for yourself based on your interests, talents, skills, and abilities and build up a large community of like-minded people. Sometimes it takes a while, but when you do this, you will have companies coming to you. I am not only willing to help you but I am also excited to help you, so contact me directly and let's make great things happen for you!

Tips to create the best opportunities for appropriate sponsorship:

1. Create a list of the companies and products you sincerely use and are most interested in representing. Research those companies or products and determine who to contact and how.

2. Contact potential sponsors and follow through until you get a definite answer, be it positive or negative. See it through.

3. Compile your awards and accomplishments in an organized fashion to present to potential sponsors to help your case.

4. Submit articles for publication. Create your own media opportunities and do your best in your competitions to build up a solid résumé and strong personal brand.

5. Don't burn any bridges in your career because word gets around in a specific industry. Negative interactions or reputation could prevent you from getting sponsored by other companies in the future.

6. Ask others who are sponsored how they went about securing sponsorship, what the details of their sponsorship are, and what you could expect for yourself. You'll learn from them and save time along the way.

7. Take advantage of your skills and marketable traits and characteristics and present those to potential sponsors outlining how it will benefit them.

8. Think creatively to approach a company with innovative ideas. This is a good way to stand out and get involved.

9. Align yourself with positive influential people who you may be able to use as references in your quest for sponsorship.

10. Research the companies you seek sponsorship from so you know a lot about them and can reference aspects of your research that you appreciate in your discourse with the company. They will respect your thoughtfulness and research efforts.

Using your body transformation to get sponsored and boost your career in the fitness industry

One of the best ways to get sponsored in the first place is the result of a well-documented body transformation. Losing a dramatic amount of weight or gaining a significant amount of muscle will not only make you feel better and look better, but open doors to a myriad of career opportunities. To see an example of this, go to www.bodybuilding.com and look at my friend Tiffany Forni's profile. Her transformation of losing over 100 pounds and becoming a fitness champion led to her sponsorship with Bodybuilding.com and many other companies. This is just one example of someone I know personally and there are thousands of other examples everywhere on websites, magazine and television advertising, and product labels.

Body transformations are extremely marketable, especially when connected to a specific product, diet, training program, or lifestyle. When you embark on a body transformation challenge, whether you are out of shape, overweight, underweight, an off-season bodybuilder, or in any other condition that you wish to change, the most important key to remember is to accurately document your progress through writing, photos, and videos with the actual dates noted. A body transformation can be useless when it comes to marketing or inspiring others if there is no evidence of it and no record to show for it. The more detailed your documentation, the better off you'll be. Date your entries and establish your goals from the beginning to show what it is that you're working toward. Take progress photos and videos all along the way.

Most of us stumble upon a body transformation out of personal desire to change, to lose weight, gain muscle, tone up, prepare to compete in a competition, or simply improve health and appearance. If being marketable and landing a sponsorship with a major company is your goal, having some sort of unique approach is going to be necessary. What makes you so special? Why choose you over all these other people? What makes you the best fit for the company? Those are some questions you are going to want to think about before you even begin a body transformation. Don't just change for the sake of changing. Have meaningful reasons behind your attempt to land yourself a sponsor based on your transformation. This will keep you focused and make success easier to attain.

If the goal is to be sponsored by a vegan product, then it would be wise to use that product during your transformation and document it in as many ways as possible. If your goal is to represent a specific diet such as a vegan diet, raw food vegan diet, or whole food-based vegan diet, you'll want to follow that lifestyle as closely as possible while charting progress. If you aspire to represent a clothing company, wear their brand when you train, travel, compete, etc. and take photos and videos to display your level of dedication, commitment and loyalty to their brand. In the natural products industry and supplement industry I see this all the time. Athletes will use a specific product or claim to use a specific product or line of products and use their success with the products as leverage to get sponsored. This is what I do for Vega as well. I used Vega products every day for three months leading up to a competition I won, which makes for a great testimonial.

When you have completed your body transformation using whatever products or services you really believe in, put your story together in an organized presentation and submit it to your target companies and organizations or media.

Once you have been selected to be sponsored by a company or organization, your work isn't over. There are likely many people who are sponsored and you will still need to find ways to stand out. One of the best ways to be successful as a sponsored athlete is simply behaving the way you would love to see someone working for you behave. If you are out-going, friendly, enthusiastic, and fun to be around, you will be well liked within your company. That should lead to a great relationship, increased sales, and future opportunities. I can't tell you how often I have been turned off by a product or company because I didn't get a good feel for the person or representative who was associated with the company during my interactions with them. This plays a major role in who I decide to support, which products I buy, and which products I decide to promote to friends and to large audiences. Subsequently, I can't tell you how often I have been impressed with certain companies based on the pleasant interaction I had with their representatives. This absolutely dictates my shopping experiences and where I invest my money. You can sincerely enjoy what you're doing or you can just go through the motions and put yourself at risk of being replaced. Being outgoing, friendly, approachable, and personable is a natural way to increase your chances of success. Some of those traits are inherent in some people but can also be learned and put into practice.

Robert's Recap on how to market yourself to get sponsored

Determine the companies you like the most and would most like to represent and create a detailed plan of action to seek their sponsorship. Use your strengths, your resources, your networks, and your own personal characteristics and attributes to earn sponsorship. Avoid the common pit-falls. Build up a strong and powerful résumé by having an intelligent work ethic. Once you become sponsored, work hard to maintain the opportunity you have in front of you and use it to build your own personal brand simultaneously.

The more you give of yourself in sincere ways to the companies you represent, the more they will give you in return. This could mean more money, more travel, more exposure, more products, and more opportunities. All of those things often lead to more fun, greater rewards, and more personal fulfillment. Don't just go the extra mile, go the extra ten miles because down the road it will pay off in amazing ways. Be the person you see in others who inspire you to be great at what you do. Be the type of person you would love to have represent your own company. Do the little things that make a big difference.

Robert's Top 10 tips to market yourself effectively to get sponsored

1. Be yourself and work hard to use your personality traits in the most productive ways to demonstrate to potential sponsors that you have the charisma they are looking for in an ambassador of their products.

2. Be persistent. If you want something badly enough, you'll be willing to work hard for it and you'll be willing to follow up and follow through until you get what you want.

3. Find a company or organization that is the best fit for you. Don't get caught up pursuing something that doesn't look like a good fit from the get go. Use your time wisely by targeting your efforts effectively.

4. Be an outstanding person. What separates you from the others? Make sure that you create an identity for yourself that is remarkable and you'll achieve outstanding results.

5. Display the fact that you really care. The more sincere and authentic you are, the better you will be perceived and the more likely you will be able to entice a sponsor to want to work with you.

6. Build up a strong résumé. Why would company X want to work with you? What do you have to offer and what does your proven track record look like?

7. Volunteer your time, resources, or efforts to contribute to the company or organization from which you seek sponsorship to demonstrate your deep interest in their products. The more you give to them the more they will give to you.

8. Keep records of those you've influenced to use as testimonials to

support the products you hope to promote and represent.

9. Build up a strong social media presence. Who knows who you are? What is the size of your following and how loyal is your community? The stronger your web presence, especially in social media and social networks, the more influence you have and the higher your market value is in the eyes and wallets of potential sponsors.

10. Use your connections, resources, and networks. Don't overlook the power of who you know.

"I operate a Natural Food Demo Company called Positive Living Products, and I started doing demos for Vega's vegan meal replacement powder three years ago when I met Robert. He was the Oregon Rep for Vega, and I was doing live demonstrations for the Vega products in stores. I can honestly say Robert has saved me as an athlete and an active business owner with his expertise and passion of plant based-athletics. Robert's dedication to a vegan lifestyle in the bodybuilding world has inspired me and hundreds at my demo tables. We all admire the muscles Robert has built on a vegan lifestyle. Many athletes that I connect with are blown away by Robert's body since no animal or dairy proteins were ingested to enhance his build. It is extraordinary. I am grateful to be a part of the Vega team and to know Robert."

Lorie Fleischman
Owner/Positive Living Products
Ashland, OR

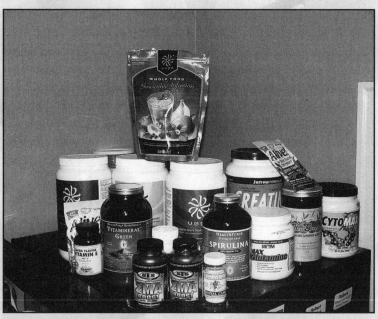

Supplements on top of Robert's refrigerator at home

Chapter 10

Supplementation – What to Take and Why

"In the next ten years, one of the things you're bound to hear is that animal protein is one of the most toxic nutrients of all that can be considered...Quite simply, the more you substitute plant foods for animal foods, the healthier you are likely to be. I now consider veganism to be the ideal diet. A vegan diet—particularly one that is low in fat— will substantially reduce disease risks. Plus, we've seen no disadvantages from veganism."

T. Colin Campbell, Ph.D.
Nutritional biochemist, Cornell University
Author of *The China Study*

The second most popular question after "how do you get your protein?" is "What supplements do you take?" There were periods of my vegan bodybuilding life when I didn't use any supplements at all and made incredible gains. But I do use supplements today, and I will share with you my favorite supplements and the most popular bodybuilding supplements for athletes, explaining what their function is and how they can benefit vegan athletes and competitive bodybuilders.

The following is a list of common bodybuilding supplements and their functions or roles in contributing to health and athletic success. Additional information about each one can easily be found through Internet searches.

Protein Powders

Protein supplements are used to enhance muscle repair and growth. Inadequate protein intake causes a negative nitrogen balance, which slows muscle growth and causes fatigue. In an athlete with normal renal function, there are no notable adverse effects to increased protein consumption.[21]

---

[21] http://www.brianmac.co.uk/drugs.htm

Protein powders come in many plant-based forms including hemp, pea, rice, soy, buckwheat, spirulina and artichoke. Protein powders are a very convenient way to increase your protein intake in an easily digested and assimilated liquid form once added to water or another liquid. If you fear you have a low protein intake, protein powders are one of the best remedies. They have also been shown to be extremely beneficial for adding muscle when consumed by bodybuilders and other athletes.

My favorite protein powders come from hemp, pea, and rice protein, namely the Vega brand products. I like pure brown rice protein and pure pea protein as well.

Protein Bars

Protein bars are conveniently packaged nutrition bars often made of nuts, seeds, fruits, and dates or agave nectar. They usually contain anywhere from 6 to 24 grams of protein per bar and vary in price based on their size, weight, and ingredient profile. Protein bars provide condensed nutrition and add more total protein and calories to your bodybuilding diet in a pleasant-tasting, easily-consumed, convenient form. They are available at not only nutrition stores and fitness centers but also in convenience stores from gas stations to college campuses all over North America.

I have many favorite bars, but the high protein Clif and Organic Food bars are among my favorites for protein content alone. I also enjoy Vega bars, Lara bars, PROBAR, and a variety of vegan bars that seem to dominate the shelves in health food stores across America.

Antioxidants

An antioxidant is any compound which has the capacity to combat oxidative damage in the body induced by free radical damage. Their promotion as substances to fight age-related damage is widespread in the popular and health related media. Although studies support their use in preventing some disease states, a number of large clinical trials cast doubt on the effectiveness of antioxidants, with some suggesting they may even do more harm than good. With so much conflicting data, the one thing that is generally agreed on is that the lower incidence of disease experienced by people eating a wide range of fruit and vegetables may have more to do with bioflavonoids in the food, rather than the role of one particular antioxidant such as Vitamin C or Vitamin E.[22]

---

[22] Stanner SA, Hughes J, Kelly CN, Buttriss J (2004). "A review of the epidemiological evidence for the 'antioxidant hypothesis'". Public Health Nutr 7 (3): 40722. http://www.brianmac.co.uk/drugs.htm

Berries and exotic fruits contain high levels of antioxidants. Some of the most popular and commonly used foods for their antioxidant content are blueberries, acaí berries, pomagranates, acerola cherries, cranberries, apples, and many Amazon fruits and a variety of beans such as kidney beans and black beans.

I personally enjoy antioxidant fruit drinks, and since fruit is my favorite type of food, it is easy and enjoyable for me to consume high antioxidant foods regularly. Sambazon and Bossa Nova are my favorite antioxidant-specific juice companies. I enjoy the quality of their products, their flavors, and the friendly staff members I've met representing their brands at various health festivals around the country.

Amino Acids

Essential Amino Acids

Did you know?: It is easy to get all the protein you need without eating meats (any animal tissue).

Did you know?: Your body gets all but 1/6 of the protein it needs from recycling old body tissue. This 1/6 must come from essential amino acids you eat.

Every cell in the body is comprised of proteins. Amino acids are the chemical substances that make up protein. Our bodies use 22 amino acids to make the 50,000 different proteins we must have to be healthy. Of the 22 amino acids there are 8 that are essential for human nutrition. An essential amino acid is one that cannot be synthesized from other available resources, and therefore must be supplied as part of the diet.

It is not important to mix plant material at one meal to obtain the 8 amino acids because our bodies store amino acids in our blood for several hours. So if we miss getting some amino acids in one meal, we can pick them up at some other time during the day. Non-essential amino acids don't need to be supplied in the diet as they can be synthesized from other dietary substances. Nearly every food, with the exception of fruits, sugars, fats and oils, has enough protein to supply our necessary amino acids if we eat enough of it to get our day's worth of calories. We do not need to eat meat.

The 8 essential amino acids are:

- Tryptophan - Tryptophan is a precursor for serotonin and melatonin. It is plentiful in chocolate, oats, bananas, dried dates, milk, cottage cheese, meat, fish, turkey, and peanuts.

- Lysine - Lysine deficiency can result in a deficiency in niacin (Vitamin B) and this can cause the disease pellagra. It is also beneficial in treating and preventing herpes. Lysine sources include green beans, lentils, soybean, spinach, and amaranth.

- Methionine - Methionine supplies sulfur and other compounds required by the body for normal metabolism and growth. It belongs to a group of compounds called lipotropics that help the liver process fats. It is found in fish, whole grains, and dairy.

- Valine - Valine is needed for muscle metabolism, tissue repair, and for the maintenance of proper nitrogen balance in the body. Valine is found in high concentration in the muscle tissue. It is also one of the three branched-chain amino acids, which means that it can be used as an energy source by muscle tissue. It may be helpful in treating liver and gallbladder disorders and it is good for correcting the type of severe amino acid deficiencies that can be caused by drug addiction. Dietary sources of valine include dairy products, grain, meat, mushrooms, peanuts, and soy proteins.

- Leucine - Leucine is a branched-chain essential amino acid that stimulates muscle protein synthesis and may be the major fuel involved in anabolic (tissue building) reactions. During times of starvation, stress, infection, or recovery from trauma, the body mobilizes leucine as a source for gluconeogenesis (the synthesis of blood sugar in the liver) to aid in the healing process. It has recently been suggested that leucine may have beneficial therapeutic effects on the prevention of protein wasting, as it occurs during starvation, semi-starvation, trauma, or recovery after surgery. Insulin deficiency is known to result in poor utilization of leucine; therefore, individuals who suffer from glucose intolerance may require higher levels of leucine intake. Leucine is found in cottage cheese, sesame seeds, peanuts, dry lentils, chicken, and fish.

- Isoleucine - Isoleucine is a branched-chain amino acid that is important for blood sugar regulation, muscle development and repair, hemoglobin development, and energy regulation. Deficiencies of isoleucine result in possible dizziness, headaches, fatigue, depression, confusion and irritability. Isoleucine is found in eggs, fish, lentils, poultry, beef, seeds, soy, wheat, almonds and dairy.

- Threonine - Threonine is important for antibody production. It can be converted into glycine and serine. Deficiencies are rare but can result in skin disorders and weakness. Dietary sources of threonine include dairy, beef, poultry, eggs, beans, nuts, and seeds.

- Phenylalanine - Phenylalanine serves in the body as a precursor to the catecholamine family of hormones. These hormones include adrenaline and noradrenaline, which are activating substances in the central and peripheral nervous systems. Deficiencies are rare but can include slowed growth, lethargy, liver damage, weakness, oedema, and skin lesions. Food sources of phenylalanine are dairy, almonds, avocados, lima beans, peanuts, and seeds.

Food Sources

Food sources of each of the essential amino acids are mentioned in the previous section describing each essential amino acid. In general terms, proteins are found primarily in meats, eggs, milk, rice, and beans, although there are also amino acids in vegetables as well. Our bodies have to break down plant or animal protein into the component amino acids and then rebuild protein—human protein. The plant or animal protein cannot be absorbed directly because these proteins have polypeptides with hundreds, or thousands, of amino acids joined in peptide bonds that have to be broken with enzymes into the single amino acids that the body can absorb and then reform into the proteins the body requires. It is more difficult for the body to break down animal protein than plant protein.

Although most of us obtain sufficient amounts of the essential amino acids in our diets, there are conditions that require our bodies to need more than they are getting. In times of physical and emotional stress, illness, injury, and surgery the body requires more amino acids than can be gained from food alone, especially when the diet is poor. Many people are turning away from a meat-based diet because of considerations for the environment, the animals, and their own health. In these situations, it is important that people educate themselves on the best ways to obtain sufficient essential amino acids. Keep in mind that heat in cooking and the conditions of processing destroy many amino acids in our food. Vegetarians and vegans often have low intakes of the amino acid lysine that is prevalent in eggs and poultry products.

If supplementation is required, it is important to establish if the body does really need more. If supplementation is required, make sure it is pharmaceutical grade or the highest quality, pure, crystalline amino acids which are best utilized by the body since they do not require digestion and are easily absorbed.[23]

---

[23] www.glisonline.com/aminoacids.php

I get most of my amino acids through food, but I also like to supplement with specific muscle-building amino acids. BCAA's seem to be some of the most important amino acids for muscle growth, which is what my sport is all about. Additionally, the amino acid L-glutamine—the most important amino acid in muscle repair, recovery, and growth—is something that I supplement with often. I buy it in large containers on its own. It is available in a variety of brands in health food and supplement stores all over North America. I also use products that already include L-glutamine such as Vega Sport Protein powder, which contains not only protein and L-glutamine but also BCAA's. A variety of the creatine products I use also contain BCAA's and L-glutamine.

Branched-chain Amino Acids (BCAA's)

Branched-chain amino acid (BCAA) is the name given to three of the eight essential amino acids needed to make protein: leucine, isoleucine, and valine. They are called branched-chain because their structure has a 'branch' off the main trunk of the molecule. The combination of these three essential amino acids makes up approximately one-third of skeletal muscle in the human body.

In order to get energy, the body can actually break down muscle to get these BCAA's. Therefore, by supplying them during or after a workout, muscles and other tissues are spared from breakdown, which occurs as a natural part of metabolism.

Leucine is the most readily oxidized BCAA and therefore the most effective at causing insulin secretion from the pancreas. It lowers elevated blood sugar levels and aids in growth hormone production. Leucine works in conjunction with the other two BCAA's to protect muscle and act as fuel for the body. They promote the healing of bones, skin, and muscle tissue and are often recommended for patients recovering from surgery. *Note: Excessively high intake of leucine may contribute to pellagra, a disease due to niacin deficiency, and may increase the amount of ammonia in the body.*

Food sources for leucine are: nuts, beans, brown rice, soy flour, and whole wheat.

Isoleucine stabilizes and regulates blood sugar and energy levels. It is also needed for hemoglobin formation. When coupled with the other two BCAA's, they enhance energy, increase endurance, and aid in the healing and repair of muscle tissue, making them a valuable tool for athletes.

After a group of healthy people received a single intravenous infusion of these amino acids, the amount of tissue breakdown that normally occurs overnight decreased by 50 percent. In another study, the muscles of a group of marathoners and cross-country runners were spared completely with a daily dose of them.

People suffering from many different mental and physical disorders have been found to have isoleucine deficiency, which can lead to symptoms similar to those of hypoglycemia.

Isoleucine can be found in foods such as rye, almonds, cashews, chickpeas, lentils, soy protein, and most seeds.

Valine is the third BCAA. It also aids in muscle metabolism, tissue repair, and the maintenance of proper nitrogen balance in the body. It may also be helpful in treating liver and gallbladder disease and is good for correcting the type of severe amino acid deficiencies which can be caused by drug addiction. However, an excessively high level of valine can lead to symptoms such as a crawling sensation in the skin and possibly cause hallucinations.

Sources for valine are: mushrooms, peanuts, grains, and soy protein.

BCAA's are a very popular supplementation for strength in athletes. It is recommended that supplemental isoleucine should always be taken with a correct balance of the other two branched-chain amino acids—approximately two milligrams each of leucine and valine for each milligram of isoleucine. Supplements that combine all three amino acids are available and can be more convenient to use.[24]

Consumption of BCAA's should be part of an on-going supplemental program to be used regularly. BCAA supplements can be found on bodybuilding.com, the world's largest supplement seller as well as at vitamin and nutrition stores all over North America. BCAA's can be found as an individual supplement or as part of another supplement such as Vega Sport Protein, for example.

Chlorella

Chlorella is a single-celled fresh-water, microscopic algae, measuring between 2 and 8 microns in diameter (1 micron is 1,000th of 1 millimeter). Chlorella cells are round in shape and almost the same size as human red blood corpuscles.

Scientifically, chlorella belongs to green micro algae. Other relatives of the chlorella family are ao-nori and kelp-like Wakame and Kombu which are also popular as food products. Chlorella is one of the oldest forms of plant life

---

[24] http://www.healthnews.com/natural-health/amino-acids/branched-chain-amino-acids-516.html

on earth. It has the highest chlorophyll content of any known plant which gives chlorella its characteristic deep green color. Unlike most plants of multi-cells, chlorella is unicellular, which means each cell is a self-sufficient organism. Though we cannot tell by the naked eye, each chlorella cell has its own organs and functions to live alone.

No other plant grows as fast as chlorella. Because of this, it has been studied extensively as a food for the future as our world population rapidly expands beyond the present day food production capacity of the earth.

Chlorella has many clinically proven health benefits. Long acclaimed for its health promoting properties, chlorella is highly regarded and well known throughout Japan. It is believed to be their number one health food supplement with over 10 million people in Japan consuming it regularly. In fact, more people in Japan take chlorella than North Americans take Vitamin C—their most popular vitamin. Chlorella, dubbed the "Green Gem of the Orient," is deserving of its reputation as the ultimate green food.

As a true, whole superfood, chlorella has the tremendous ability to detoxify, energize, nourish, and ultimately balance all of the body's systems for optimal function.[25]

A very interesting and inspiring article about chlorella can be found on the Natural News website: http://www.naturalnews.com/026147_chlorella_cancer_blood.html.

Like most of the supplements described in this chapter, chlorella can be found at most health food stores and is available in tablets and powder form from companies such as Sequel Naturals, for example. It is also included in other supplements as an ingredient used for its cleansing and detoxifying properties and its protein and chlorophyll content. It's the food that contains the highest amounts of DNA and RNA and rebuilds itself faster than any other plant microorganism, which has great benefits to athletes when consumed after exercise.

Creatine

Unlike most supplements that athletes use, creatine is not a vitamin, mineral, herb, or hormone. It is a naturally occurring amino acid that is found in the body that has the chemical name methyl guanidine-acetic acid. Amino acids are the building blocks of proteins. The majority of creatine (about 95%) is located in the skeletal muscle system, and the remaining 5% is in the brain, heart, and testes. Humans acquire most of the creatine in the system

---

[25] http://sequelnaturals.com/chloressence/about-chlorella/botanical.html

by consuming meats and fish as well as dairy products, egg whites, nuts, and seeds. Although the human body has a way of storing very high amounts of creatine to enhance recovery and muscle power, it is quite challenging to consume enough food to provide the same amount of creatine that using supplements will. In the event that you do not consume enough creatine to suit your body's requirements, your body can synthesize it from the amino acids arginine, glycine, and methionine. This manufacturing process takes place in the kidneys, liver and pancreas.[26]

Creatine fuels ATP development, which means:

- Sustained high intensity and power workouts
- More energy for muscle contraction
- Vastly improved power and muscle size
- You workout longer, stronger, and get to see the results in the mirror.[27]

I have been using creatine off and on for ten years and have noticed that this supplement requires consistent use to produce results. If you just use creatine every once in a while, it is not likely to do much, but if you consume creatine regularly and are consistent and accountable with your supplementation, you will achieve the most noticeable results in the fastest time. Creatine is the supplement that allows me to gain the most weight and get the strongest. I know a big part of that is the retention of water weight, but being heavier allows me to lift heavier weights and I become stronger as a result. Muscle is also 70% water so I have no problem with the retention of water unless I am weeks away from a competition, in which case I discontinue use of creatine so I can drop water weight to make weight for competition and to have the leanest, driest physique on stage.

There are lots of brands of creatine available anywhere and it is also extremely affordable today compared to the cost 10-15 years ago. Nearly all creatine available is lab-made and vegan. There are varieties of creatine in both powder and liquid form with various components including creatine monohydrate, creatine citrate, creatine phosphate, creatine malate, and creatine ester. The primary difference between these types of creatine is simply what the creatine molecule is bound to, be it water (monohydrate) or malic acid (malate). Creatine monohydrate seems to be the most popular form of creatine available, though I have found it to be rough on my stomach at times

---

[26] http://www.creatine.com/en/news/2007/03/01/guarana-extract-5/
[27] http://www.creatinejournal.com/

and often use an ester form of creatine, which seems to be easier for my body to digest and reduces the bloating I get from monohydrate.

In general, I regard creatine as one of my top five supplement recommendations for those interested in building muscle and getting stronger.

Digestive Enzymes

Digestion enzymes are enzymes that break down polymeric macromolecules into smaller building blocks. Digestive enzymes are found in the digestive tract of animals (including humans) where they aid in the digestion of food as well as inside cells. Enzymes are also found in saliva, which are made from the salivary glands.

Digestive enzymes digest foods and then send the nourishing ingredients to the bloodstream to feed the organs, glands, cells, tissues, and brain. Many scientists believe that most "lifestyle" and degenerative diseases, and even aging itself, are simply the lack of a continued and adequate supply of the necessary enzymes required to keep all of the body's systems working properly.

You may be eating healthy food, but if your digestive enzymes aren't getting those nutrients to your bloodstream, organs, and cells, then you aren't receiving all the benefits of that healthy diet. Those nutrients are what keep all of your systems, particularly your immune system, strong and healthy.[28]

Digestive enzymes have played a role in my diet for years. With high consumption of soy protein foods and other foods that can be difficult to break down, assistance from enzymes is greatly appreciated to combat bloating. Enzymes are easy to find in any health food store and are not just for athletes. Enzymes can aid in anyone's ability to retain more of the nutrition they are consuming. Look for brands from natural product companies and try taking some digestive enzymes before your meal or during your meal to reduce the risk of stomach aches from foods that are difficult to break down naturally. Even natural whole foods like certain green vegetables can be very hard for the body to break down. Digestive enzymes can play a helpful role in this process.

I have used Digest Gold from Enzymedica and Digestive Enhancement Enzymes from Healthforce Nutritionals and enjoy both brands. Like the use of creatine, consistency can be another key with the consumption of enzymes. If you only use them every once in a while, you may not be able to see or feel the benefit and may not give them a sufficient try. Stick with consistent use of enzymes to enhance your absorption of nutrition and to aid in the digestion of food.

---

[28] http://www.enzymeessentials.com/HTML/enzyme_index.html

Essential Fatty Acids

Essential fatty acids, or EFAs, are fatty acids that cannot be constructed within an organism (generally all references are to humans) from other components by any known chemical pathways, and therefore must be obtained from the diet. The term refers to fatty acids involved in biological processes and not those which may just play a role as fuel. As many of the compounds created from essential fatty acids can be taken directly in the diet, it is possible that the amounts required in the diet (if any) are overestimated. It is also possible they can be underestimated as organisms can still survive in non-ideal, malnourished conditions.

There are two families of EFAs: omega-3 and omega-6. Fats from each of these families are essential, as the body can convert one omega-3 to another omega-3, for example, but cannot create an omega-3 from omega-6 or saturated fats. They were originally designated as Vitamin F when they were discovered as essential nutrients in 1923. In 1930, work by Burr, Burr and Miller showed that they are better classified with the fats than with the vitamins.[29]

Almost all the polyunsaturated fat in the human diet is from EFA. Some of the food sources of omega-3 and omega-6 fatty acids are fish and shellfish, flaxseed (linseed), hemp oil, soya oil, canola oil, chia seeds, pumpkin seeds, sunflower seeds, leafy vegetables, and walnuts.[30]

Essential fats are hugely important in the diet for everyone, as their name suggests, but play an especially important role for athletes. Consumption of essential fats makes skin and nails stronger, reduces inflammation, therefore speeds up recovery process, allowing for more frequent training. They play important roles in brain function and even help the body burn fat by affecting metabolism.

When I am preparing for a bodybuilding competition, I make a deliberate effort to consume more essential fats to help me burn body fat. I use Vega Omega 3-6-9 Essential Fatty Acid Oil Blend on salads or vegetables, and I also use Barlean's Omega Swirl and drink it straight out of the bottle. I incorporate high omega-3 and omega-6 foods into my diet all throughout the year. Some great sources for essential fats include walnuts, hempseeds, flax seeds, chia seeds, and many nuts, seeds and seed oils in general. Consume a couple of servings of omega-3 and 6-rich foods daily and you'll be well on

---

[29] Burr, G.O., Burr, M.M. and Miller, E. (1930). "On the nature and role of the fatty acids essential in nutrition" (PDF). *J. Biol. Chem.* **86** (587). http://www.jbc.org/cgi/reprint/97/1/1.pdf. Retrieved on 2007-01-17.
[30] http://en.wikipedia.org/wiki/Essential_fatty_acid

your way to improved health in many areas of life. The ideal ratio for consumption of omega-6 to omega-3 is 2:1, getting the essential fats from quality sources. Many EFA oil products have various ratios, some over-compensating with loads of Omega-3 EFAs due to the fact that people consume far more omega-6 than 3. Ideally you want to consume 5,000mg of omega-6 EFAs and 2500mg of omega-3 EFAs daily. Make sure they come from high quality sources and consume them consistently

Glutamine

Glutamine is the most abundant amino acid (building block of protein) in the bloodstream. It is considered a "conditionally essential amino acid" because it can be manufactured in the body, but under extreme physical stress, the demand for glutamine exceeds the body's ability to make it. Most glutamine in the body is stored in muscles followed by the lungs, where much of the glutamine is manufactured. Glutamine is important for removing excess ammonia (a common waste product in the body). In the process of picking up ammonia, glutamine donates it when needed to make other amino acids, as well as sugar, and the antioxidant glutathione.

Several types of important immune cells rely on glutamine for energy. Without glutamine, the immune system would not function appropriately. Glutamine also appears to be necessary for normal brain function and digestion.

Adequate amounts of glutamine are generally obtained through diet alone because the body is also able to make glutamine on its own. Certain medical conditions, including injuries, surgery, infections, and prolonged stress, can deplete glutamine levels, however. In these cases, glutamine supplementation may be helpful.

When the body is stressed (such as from injuries, infections, burns, trauma, or surgical procedures), steroid hormones, such as cortisol, are released into the bloodstream. Elevated cortisol levels can deplete glutamine stores in the body. Since glutamine plays a key role in the immune system, a deficiency in this nutrient can significantly slow the healing process. Clinical studies have reported that glutamine supplements enhance the immune system and reduce infections (particularly infections associated with surgery). Glutamine supplements may also aid in the recovery of severe burns.

Athletes who train excessively may deplete their glutamine stores. This is because they are overusing their skeletal muscles, where much of the glutamine in the body is stored. Athletes who overstress their muscles (without adequate time for recovery between workouts) may have lowered immunity and may be at increased risk for infection or slow recovery from injuries. This is also true for people who participate in prolonged exercise, such as ultra-marathon runners. For this select group of athletes, glutamine supplementation may be useful. This is not true, however, for most exercisers who tend to work out at a much more moderate intensity.

Dietary sources of glutamine include plant and animal proteins such as beef, pork, poultry, milk, yogurt, ricotta cheese, cottage cheese, raw spinach, raw parsley, and cabbage. Glutamine, usually in the form of L-glutamine, is available as an individual supplement or as part of a protein supplement. These come in powder, capsule, tablet, or liquid form.

Standard preparations are typically available in 500 mg tablets or capsules. For adults ages 18 and older, doses of 500 mg 1 to 3 times daily are generally considered safe. Doses as high as 5,000 mg to 15,000 mg daily (in divided doses) may be prescribed by a health care provider.[31]

L-glutamine is one of my all-time favorite supplements to assist with my bodybuilding program. I've been using L-glutamine for ten years and it has been a great addition to my muscle building program and effectively supports the hard work I do in the gym. Like creatine, L-glutamine is also readily available and easily accessible in stores all over North America for affordable prices. L-glutamine is a great supplement to help keep your immune system strong, your muscles growing, your body nourished and should be something you should consider including in your daily post-workout drink.

I use Techline L-glutamine or other small brands supporting growing companies and also get 4.5 grams of L-glutamine in each full serving of Vega Sport Protein. I prefer to consume a high dosage of L-glutamine every day, sometimes as high as 20 to 25 grams (20,000mg-25,000mg), typically immediately 5-10 grams after weight training or other exercise and occasionally an additional time during the day in conjunction with a protein drink or other supplement drink.

Maca

Maca is an annual plant which produces a radish-like root. The root of maca is typically dried and stored and will easily keep for seven years. The plant is cultivated in the Junin plateau of Peru's Central Highlands and was highly revered by the Inca.

During the height of the Incan empire, legend has it that Incan warriors would consume maca before entering into battle. This would make them

---

[31] http://www.umm.edu/altmed/articles/glutamine-000307.htm

fiercely strong. But after conquering a city, the Incan soldiers were prohibited from using maca to protect the conquered women from their powerful sexual impulses. Thus as far back as 500 years ago, maca's reputation for enhancing strength, libido, and fertility was already well established in Peru.

Today, maca's popularity is very much on the increase, as people discover that the plant really does boost libido, sexual function, and overall energy. Acreage in Peru dedicated to Maca cultivation is increasing every year to meet demand, and a number of scientists have turned their attention to the properties of the root. In Peru, maca is used by men and by women who want to put more fire into their sex lives. And in the U.S., Europe, and Japan, dietary supplements containing maca are gaining ardent devotees.

In-depth analysis of maca conducted in 1998 by Dr. Qun Yi Zheng and his colleagues at PureWorld Botanicals shows that maca contains about 10 percent protein, almost 60 percent carbohydrate, and an assortment of fatty acids.[32]

The growing demand of the supplement industry has been one of the primary reasons for maca's expansion. The prominent product is maca flour, which is ground from the hard, dried roots. In Peru, maca flour is used in baking as a base and a flavoring. The supplement industry uses both the dry roots and maca flour for different types of processing and concentrated extracts. Maca is one of many root vegetables with a dense fiber matrix which can be gelatinized to create products with more efficient digestion. Gelatinized maca is many times stronger than powdered root and is employed mainly for therapeutic, medicinal, and supplement purposes. It can also be used like maca flour. There is also freeze-dried maca juice, which is a juice squeezed from the macerated fresh root and subsequently freeze-dried.[33]

I learned about maca five years ago and have been using it ever since. Don't be thrown off by the word "gelatin" in *gelatinized*. It doesn't contain any animal products but is simply the name for the process for removing starchy carbohydrates from the plant. Maca comes in a variety of forms including powders and vegicaps. There are a variety of brands producing maca these days and Sequel Naturals is the brand I use the most. Visit any health food store to get your own container of maca. It will help nourish your adrenal glands which help you combat stress and enable you to perform better,

---

[32] http://health.discovery.com/centers/sex/libido/maca.html

[33] Skyfield Tropical: Free Online Botanical Encyclopedia "http://www.skyfieldtropical.com/encyclopedia/maca/" Maca (lepidium peruvianum): Botanical Characteristics (Courtesy of http://en.wikipedia.org/wiki/Lepidium_meyenii).

train better, and recover from exercise sufficiently so you can train even more effectively.

Meal Replacement Powders

Meal replacement powders (MRP's) or shakes are nutritionally complete products designed to contain required nutrients the body needs daily. They contain complete protein, carbohydrates, fats and essential fatty acids, amino acids, vitamins, minerals, and digestive enzymes. Some have other characteristics too, such as prebiotics, probiotics, antioxidants, and "super foods."

MRP's are convenient and increasingly popular as people become busier. The only thing required is some sort of container and liquid. Usually a water bottle filled with water will do the trick nicely. Most are already flavored and will not need to be blended or have other ingredients added to them, though other foods could be added to enhance texture or taste. They are designed to be ready to consume with added water when they come in powder form. Others are already in ready-to-drink packaging for immediate consumption.

I have been using Vega for nearly half a decade and it has been a huge part of my bodybuilding nutrition program. Vega is a plant-based, common allergen-free meal replacement powder that not only has protein but also 100% RDI vitamins and minerals, essential fats, digestive enzymes, antioxidants, and many other components, including containing maca and chlorella.

MRP's are the one supplement I promote the most and encourage others to use the most. Simply, they cover everything from protein to fats to vitamins to antioxidants and to me that makes them more effective than any individual supplement. Use MRP's as a breakfast, a snack, or a post-workout shake to get the nutrition you need to keep growing.

Pre-workout drinks

Pre-workout drinks are full of sugars and carbohydrates to stimulate the body and increase energy to aid in a productive workout or exercise session. They typically include easily digested carbohydrates, caffeine, and other stimulants like ginseng, yerba maté, green tea, and nitric oxide.

Most pre-workout drinks are designed to be consumed 30 minutes before a workout and during a workout for continued energy.

Currently I'm using Vega Sport Performance Optimizer pre-workout powder which is an all-natural performance enhancer specializing in assisting the body with energy, stamina, mental focus, and recovery through its purpose-driven ingredients that even aid in reducing inflammation after exercise. I also use the electrolyte drink Ultima Replenisher during some of my workouts and enjoy the flavors and energy benefits.

In general, I use pre-workout drinks more often than almost any other supplement. I enjoy having the pre-workout drinks during my workouts as well as immediately before, and whether it is a green tea beverage or a sports-specific supplement, I'm normally drinking something before and during training sessions to give myself an extra boost. I like the psychological benefit of having the pump-up drink with me during my workout. I like the extra calories that fuel my workout all the way through, and I like the opportunity to put more liquid in my diet, especially during a time when I'm losing fluids through sweating.

Recovery drinks

Recovery drinks are often filled with carbohydrates to replace depleted glycogen stores and also contain amino acids and protein to aid in muscle repair, recovery, and growth. Recovery drinks may also contain nutrients lost through exercise such as sodium, magnesium, and potassium eliminated from the body through sweat. Many recovery drinks are forms of meal replacement or protein powders since a major part of recovery is the amino acids needed for muscle repair. It is usually recommended to consume a recovery drink within an hour of your exercise session, and some people, including myself, like to take a recovery drink immediately following exercise during the post-workout nutritional window of opportunity to get the muscle repair process started right away.

Other popular components of a recovery drink include creatine and essential fats. I often create my own unique mixtures using a protein powder with creatine and L-glutamine added to it. Sometimes I'll combine multiple protein powders like Sun Warrior and Vega to get a mixture of flavors, textures, and a mixed amino acid profile. The Vega Sport Protein is designed to contain protein, BCAA's, and L-glutamine which makes it an all natural recovery powder that is ready to go with added water. Discover which products are your favorites and focus on consuming a recovery drink immediately after your workout or within 30 to 60 minutes afterward for best results.

Vitamins

Vitamins are found naturally in foods, especially fruits. Vitamins play a lot of roles in our health including some of the obvious roles like supporting and boosting our immune system and helping us stay healthy and strong. They also play some very specific roles. In bodybuilding a variety of vitamins stand out including Vitamin C, Vitamin E, and Vitamin B-12. Improved immune system, brain function and muscle function are goals of bodybuilders and should be goals for anyone, and these key vitamins contribute substantially to improved health and athletic performance.

I always encourage everyone to take some sort of multivitamin or a meal replacement which acts as a multivitamin daily. Because we don't always eat as much of a variety of plant-based whole foods as we think we do, it benefits us to ensure we are getting all vitamins by taking a quality multivitamin supplement. As usual, look for the most natural brands, and products that are found at quality health food stores rather than common grocery stores. Popular quality brands include New Chapter, NOW, and Country Life. There are many other natural smaller brands so check with your local quality vitamin retailer or community health food store for additional options.

A list of vitamins and their functions is the following:

Vitamin B1 (thiamin)
Enhances energy production, increases aerobic capacity, improves concentration

Vitamin B2 (riboflavin)
Increases aerobic endurance

Vitamin B6 (pyridoxine)
Enhances muscle growth, decreases anxiety

Vitamin B12 (cyanocobalamin)
Enhances muscle growth

Vitamin B15 (dimethylglycine)
Increases muscle energy production

Vitamin C
Acts as antioxidant, increases aerobic capacity and energy production

Vitamin E
Acts as antioxidant, improves aerobic capacity[34]

---

[34] http://www.brianmac.co.uk/drugs.htm

List of Robert's Favorite Supplements

Protein Powders

Vega Sport Protein Powder (hemp, pea, rice, spirulina, alfalfa juice proteins with BCAA's, L-glutamine, and digestive enzymes) – www.myvega.com

Vega Smoothie Infusion (hemp, pea, rice protein with greens) – www.myvega.com

Sun Warrior (brown rice protein) – www.sunwarrior.com

Pure Advantage Pea Protein (pea protein) - http://www.pureadvantage.net/protein_powder_pure_pea_ protein.asp

Protein/Energy Bars

Vega Bars – www.myvega.com

PROBAR – www.theprobar.com

Clif Builder Bars – www.clifbar.com

Organic Food Bars – www.organicfoodbar.com

Lara Bars – www.larabar.com

Meal Replacement Powders

Vega Whole Food Health Optimizer – www.myvega.com

Pre-Workout Supplements

Vega Sport Performance Optimizer pre-workout powder – www.myvega.com

Ultima Replenisher - www.ultimareplenisher.com

Other Supplement Favorites:

Techline L-glutamine – www.eliteathleteinc.com

Techline Creatine - www.eliteathleteinc.com

Vega omega 3-6-9 EFA Oil – www.myvega.com

Barlean's Omega Swirl - www.barleans.com/omega_swirl.asp

Sambazon antioxidant drinks – www.sambazon.com

Guayaki Yerba Maté drinks – www.guayaki.com

Himalaya Herbal Healthcare supplements – www.himalayausa.com

Healthforce Nutritionals all natural vegan supplements – www.healthforce.com

*For a complete list of *vegan* supplements available for purchase visit www.veganessentials.com

If I could only suggest five supplements to help with bodybuilding success they would be:

1. Meal Replacement powders
2. Protein Powders
3. BCAA's
4. L-glutamine
5. Creatine

Normally I would have a multivitamin on that list, but a meal replacement covers multivitamins as well. If you simply use two or three of the top five supplements, you will enhance your bodybuilding program and achieve greater success. If you use all five, you'll achieve ultimate success in muscle building. The bottom line is, consuming whole foods should be your primary objective in health and wellness and bodybuilding nutrition, but the use of supplements speeds up success and acts just as the name suggests, supplementing your nutrition program. Supplements can get expensive so pick out the ones that give you the greatest benefits based on your health and fitness goals and use them to supplement your sound nutrition program. Work hard to get sponsored by products you truly use and enjoy to cut down on your supplement expenses. Your sound nutrition and supplementation programs combined with your exercise program will become the foundation of your achievement and something you can always count on as you progress and take this lifestyle and sport as far as you want to take it.

Robert's Recap of Supplementation describing what to take and why

Some of the greatest years of my bodybuilding life were without the use of supplements, but there is no doubt that the BEST periods of my bodybuilding career were supported by supplementation, namely from protein powders in general—Vega products, L-glutamine, Nitric Oxide, and Creatine. Like any other aspect of bodybuilding, I've determined that the most important factor in success with supplementation is consistency. Consistently using supplements appropriately really gives the body an opportunity to adapt with the extra fire power it has to work with, and that makes for a more successful bodybuilding career. Use products that are as natural as possible. There are plenty of vegan supplements that are filled with dyes and chemicals and many other agents that are not nearly as natural as they could be. Vega Sport Performance Optimizer is much more natural than BSN's NO Explode, for example. They are different in their make-up but are both pre-workout powders designed to fuel the workout to make it better.

Focus on the basics to get the best results. Nothing beats protein powders, meal replacement powders, L-glutamine, essential fats, vitamin/mineral supplements, BCAA's, and creatine. These are the basics to provide the best results to enhance your bodybuilding lifestyle. Ask others for advice on which supplements they are taking and what their experiences have been. Call the companies and ask questions, including confirming that no animal products were used and no animals were tested on. Try a variety of natural supplements and document your experiences with them for future references. Be safe and take the recommended dosages of the supplements you use.

Robert's Top 10 tips for Supplementation on a Vegan Bodybuilding diet

1. Stick with the basics: protein, vitamins, amino acids, essential fats, and creatine.

2. Read supplement reviews and talk with others who have used the supplements you are interested in using.

3. Don't give up on a supplement if you haven't given it a fair shot with consistent use. Some products take longer to show their benefits and results than others.

4. When you see others at your gym thriving in their bodybuilding career, ask them what supplements they are taking and determine if they fit your interests and are supplements you may want to incorporate into your program as well.

5. Read labels to confirm the supplements you're interested in are vegan-friendly or vegan-approved. Use websites such as www.veganessentials.com, www.foodfightgrocery.com, and www.veganproteins.com as resources since 100% of the supplements on their websites are certified or confirmed vegan.

6. If you have questions about a specific supplement, join an online discussion board to pose questions for a diverse audience, or call the company directly.

7. Remember that nothing replaces the nutrition from whole foods in their natural state, but when you don't have access to a lot of fresh and local whole foods, supplements are a great way to give your nutrition program a boost.

8. Document your results using supplements in a journal so you have an accurate record of your usage and experiences that you can review later and share with others.

9. Create a budget for supplements because they are a cost that can quickly add up in a bodybuilding lifestyle. Don't overlook this aspect of budgeting and planning or you could end up with financial troubles as a result of your desire to improve your physique.

10. As often as possible, use the supplements that are the most natural and have the least amount of potential side-effects. It's always better to stick to natural supplements whenever possible so you have a better idea of what you're putting in your body.

"One year ago I had the incredible opportunity to live with Robert Cheeke. My athletic background was in endurance sports with an attitude of not wanting to lift weights. But that all changed after only six months of living with Robert. With his encouragement and inspiration, I was instantly hooked on lifting weights in the weight room. As of today, I am training for my first fitness model competition. I owe it all to Robert Cheeke!

Robert has been working his whole life to get to where he is. I learned from him that it takes a lot of planning, staying positive, hard work, determination, and dedication to get where you want to go in life. Robert is good at what he does, and you can honestly see it in his eyes that he loves what he does."

Natasha West
Friend, Organic Athlete member, VeganBodybuilding.com member
Victoria, B.C.

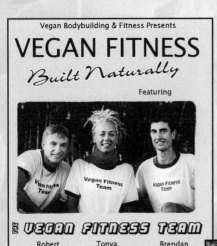

DVD cover for the documentary
Vegan Fitness Built Naturally (2005)

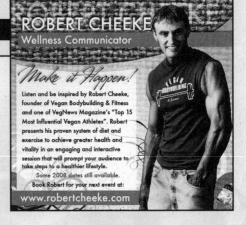

Robert's first paid advertising
feature in VegNews Magazine
for a speaking tour in 2008

Chapter 11

Turning your Passion into a Career

"If one advances confidently in the directions of his dreams, and endeavors to live the life which he has imagined, he will meet with a success unexpected in common hours."

Henry David Thoreau
American author, poet, naturalist

What if you could turn your passion into your career, would you do it? In other words, if you could pick your favorite things in the world to do and get paid adequately to do them every day, would you be interested? I have a feeling your answer is, "yes" without hesitation. Who wouldn't want to get paid to do what they already love to do? I don't know many people who would pass up that opportunity. But the truth is, most of us pass up this opportunity everyday of our lives. There are interests in our lives that we enjoy so much we would pay to do them. There are interests that if pursued properly would enable us to do them all the time and in fact get paid to do so.

What if I told you that turning a dream into reality is easier than you think; would you be up for it? What if I told you that it is not only a possibility but can be an extremely rewarding real-life scenario that can lead to the greatest times of your life; would you be in?

It is my experience that if you truly love something, you will be willing to spend a lot of time doing it, will be willing to work harder than others to achieve it, and will have so much fun throughout the process that you will excel naturally. The joy and fulfillment you get from being regularly engaged in the activity you love will propel you to stand out in your field, adapting and improving at rapid rates. You will look forward to practice, rehearsal, application, and action in whatever it is that moves you. Through your discipline and dedication, you will thrive in an environment you created that is perfect for you to succeed in. Because you're doing what you love, you'll be in a positive mood on a regular basis, will find the good in every situation, will get back up when you're knocked down, and will time and time again overcome adversity where others with less passion will give in and give up. Regardless of what your passion in life is, I am confident that you can turn it into a successful lifestyle, a fulfilling career, and one of the most rewarding areas of your life you have ever experienced.

You can check out my step-by-step equation for success in any area of life in my 300-page book *Take Action and Make it Happen – Bringing out the Best in You*. The entire book is dedicated to that concept and is more practical and more detailed than any other I have seen on the subject. My *Take Action and Make it Happen* book should be released in late 2010 or early 2011. I mention this concept in *this* book and even have this chapter dedicated to it in order to help you specifically turn your passion for veganism or fitness or both into a career. There are plenty of career opportunities that vegan athletes are typically drawn to, and I'm outlining and describing some of them here and providing some insight on how to get started on them and put them into action immediately.

I turned my passion for vegan bodybuilding into a career when I formed my own business Vegan Bodybuilding & Fitness back in 2002 and launched my website www.veganbodybuilding.com in 2003, released my clothing line in 2003, my first documentary in 2005, and my first published book in 2010. I accomplished a lot of things that on paper wouldn't look very probable. I don't have a college degree and spent less than a year in college, but I run my own company, have been the number one salesperson in the country for multiple companies, have produced an award-winning documentary, produced a second documentary that is sure to win some awards, have secured a literary agent in New York, acquired a Public Relations Manager, and have written three 300-page books over the past 18 months while becoming one of the top public speakers in my entire industry touring North America for the past three years. I will also make a six-figure income this year doing exactly what I want to do in life, enjoying seven days a week, not just the weekends. None of those things I accomplished were "supposed" to happen for me. I'm not well educated scholastically. I've never had a lot of money. In fact, I have been relatively poor my entire life, especially my entire adult life, and I have a lot of personal issues in my life battling situations that impact me mentally and emotionally on a daily basis. Looking at my education, qualifications, and experiences on paper wouldn't reflect an innovative, creative, and bright future pioneering a modern era of an entire movement, but there is something that can't be seen or measured on paper, and that is heart, will, desire, and unwavering persistence. Those things I had more than sufficient supply of, and that is precisely what propelled me to the top of my industry and allowed me to make a dream a reality and turn my passion into an incredible career that is really just taking off.

The lesson to be learned is that we need not sell ourselves short based on perceived limitations. I never expected to fail or underachieve because I wasn't as smart as someone else who was working toward a similar goal. I always believed in my ability to be outstanding, and it was my firm, sincere belief in myself that made me exceptional and made success a reality rather than an unattainable destination I feared I'd never see. I knew what I wanted to get out of life, and I went after it with all my heart. I was willing to put it all on the line because I learned from role models who did the same.

The greatest role model in my life is a man I never met, a man who died before I was born, but who left a lasting impression on me that changed my life forever. My greatest hero is America's Greatest Running Legend Steve Prefontaine (Pre). Pre was determined to test the limits of the human heart through the passion, effort, and love he had not only for his sport but also for being his best and for being the world's very best. He demonstrated a self-expression of pure will and courage that is greater than any expression of heart I have ever witnessed. It was Pre's influence on me when I was 18 years old that gave me the courage and confidence that I could do anything in the world and that I could be the best in the world. By time I reached the age he died, which was 24 years old, I was the best in the world at what I was doing and have not let up ever since because Pre wouldn't have let up either. He would have pushed it as far as his heart, lungs, and body would have allowed him to push until he had absolutely nothing left. That is how I am living my life—without limits, in honor of one of the greatest role models our world has ever seen. If you're inspired or moved to learn more about Steve Prefontaine, please look for one or all of three movies made about him, *Without Limits*, *Prefontaine*, and the documentary *Fire on the Track*. A book was also written about his life called *Pre: The Story of America's Greatest Running Legend, Steve Prefontaine*, written by Tom Jordan. You can also do your own research online. The moment I met Pre's parents in 1999, my life changed forever in the most amazing ways, just from the one day I spent with them learning about their son, and I owe a lot of my success to Steve Prefontaine's influence. Of course it wasn't solely Pre's influence on me that made me great at what I was doing, but it was a major factor and worth mentioning to make the point that a role model can have a major impact on your success. By understanding that you can see that as a role model yourself, you can have that type of powerful influence on others too, and that is one of the greatest feelings in life; to genuinely inspire other people to believe in themselves.

So what if you're like me and you don't exactly have the best résumé to get your career off to a flying start? Well, you do what anyone needs to do if they hope to excel at something: believe in your abilities wholeheartedly; apply yourself deliberately; dig deep into your heart to fuel your passion to become great. Anyone can do it; you just have to find what matters most in your life and apply a series of principles sequentially. If you do this, success naturally follows.

Despite my lack of formal higher education, I have been able to accomplish more than most, just in my 20's. I'm not afraid to admit my lack of education, though I had spent the past ten years being embarrassed about it. I found solace in the fact that some of my other role models also dropped out of college and made great careers for themselves following their own passions, heart, and desires while being innovative, creative, and pioneers of their industries such as Steve Jobs from Apple and Bill Gates from Microsoft. I have plenty of other role models who are very well educated including bestselling authors Richard Dawkins, Sam Harris, Christopher Hitchens, and Daniel Dennett among many other scholars and intellects. The truth is that I never felt comfortable addressing my lack of education because I didn't think I had accomplished enough on my own to make up for it. Even with my own company, my status at the most recognized vegan bodybuilder in the world, having an award-winning documentary that I wrote, directed, produced, and starred in, I wasn't confident enough to openly talk about my limited education. Then I followed my own advice, my inherent belief in my ability to succeed in any new project. I wrote three books that are 1,000 combined pages, which will all become best-sellers in the way that everything else I do turns into success because of the actions I take to ensure it. When I completed my second book, I had it accepted by a literary agent in New York and presented to the largest book publishers in the world. My confidence grew, even when I was rejected by the publishers I dreamed of having publish my book. I remained confident because, like I do so often throughout my life when I get rejected or hit obstacles, I resolved to make my books best-sellers even if I have to do it my own way and without large corporate support. Once again, I will prove that heart doesn't always show up on paper, but pushing the limits of my own heart is what makes me prevail time and time again, no matter what my aspirations are. This will be no different. My resilience makes me a lot more dangerous, adversity makes me bite back harder, and obstacles make me climb over more people to get to my desired destination. This never-give-up approach is exactly what it takes to turn your passion into a career. You can do it in any industry by being the most mentally tough person anyone has ever seen. You can do it in the vegan bodybuilding and fitness industry by following my lead and my example of drive, passion, grit, and determination; or you can create your own path and do it all your own way on your own terms, calling the shots, and being in charge of your own destiny.

There are countless possible outcomes, and failure isn't one of them. You have to understand that right now. If you aren't willing to understand that, then put this book down right now and find something else to do and read my other personal development books to find out why success matters. If you expect failure, fear failure, or make yourself susceptible and vulnerable to failure, you open yourself up to failure. That isn't an option if you truly care enough to succeed. When you accept, just like I did, that you are not limited by your education, your experiences, your résumé, your age, size, or gender but that you are capable and have more heart and more guts than anyone else, you are not only ready for success, but you are on the path to attaining it doing something you absolutely love to do.

In this book I want to specifically address finding a career within the vegan bodybuilding and fitness industry. You're reading this book for a reason. Likely, it is because you have some sort of interest in veganism or athletics, and you may be considering a career involving one or both of the industries. So, what's it going to be? What about this industry makes you want to learn more about it, and what makes you want to be part of it? What are you going to do with your life to be able to say, "I have the best job in the world for me?" What are you going to invest in and sacrifice so you can look forward to Monday, Tuesday, Wednesday, Thursday, Friday, Saturday, and Sunday rather than just the weekends? You know my unlikely story of going from skinny farm boy to the world's most recognized vegan bodybuilder. What story are you going to tell? How will you become the type of role model I have been for many and the type of role model Steve Prefontaine has been for me? I am excited to hear your answers to these questions, and I'm even more excited to watch your success develop before my eyes.

There are plenty of careers available to those of us in the vegan fitness industry and many careers that we make for ourselves. None of my careers had titles. There weren't job openings or listings for vegan fitness documentary producers. I just went out and did it. There weren't openings at the local book publishing houses looking for literary work about vegans lifting weights. I created the opportunity on my own. There certainly wasn't a job posting for a vegan to go around the country visiting Universities flexing and motivating students to be extraordinary, but I did it anyway. That is the type of creativity and innovation that can take you from average to outstanding if only you are willing to do what it takes to get there.

Some of the types of jobs that seem to be synonymous with vegan body-building and fitness or common with an aspect of those various industries are the following:

-Business Owner
-Speaker
-Author
-Fitness Model
-Spokesperson
-Company Representative
-Professional athlete
-Personal Trainer
-Nutrition store owner
-Posing Coach
-Nutrition Coach
-Product Formulator
-Outreach Coordinator
-Organization Leader
-Non-profit creator
-Website Designer
-Online Web-store owner
-Photographer
-Video Editor
-Event Organizer
-Strength and Conditioning Coach
-Actor
-Literary Agent or Editor
-Movie Producer
-Social Media Guru
-Radio Show Host
-Television Show Host
-Blogger

Some of these are general careers, but many of them are ones that vegans and vegan athletes seem to be drawn to based on their passions, interests, and lifestyle. Review the list to see if anything jumps out at you; and of course, more important than anything is to make your own list based on what you really want to do. When you discover what that is for you, pursue it with all the passion and enthusiasm in the world and accomplish great things.

If you subscribe to the belief system that you really can do anything, you will live the most incredible life because the pursuit and the journey to your eventual destination will be an experience unique only to those who dare to chase dreams. Welcome to the club. I'm a proud member and wouldn't have it any other way.

The basic model I followed to turn my passion into a career was simple. I discovered what I really wanted to do, created a detailed vision for what it would look like, and worked harder than anyone I knew to accomplish what I set out to do. I also enjoyed it. I truly loved what I was doing. I found meaning in what I was doing every step of the way, so rather than each step being a challenging one or a difficult one to muster the energy to pursue, I looked forward to each step. With that attitude I succeeded around every corner. I also practiced something that I still practice today. I could clearly visualize what the future would look like for me even when it was years off in the distance. As a skinny young kid in the gym, I pictured myself as the muscular person that I wanted to be. That inspired me through workouts moving light weights that turned to heavier weights as I improved. I could actually see myself in bodybuilding magazines years before I ended up in millions of magazine issues. I saw myself being successful, and I kept that vision in my head and worked toward it every day until I made it a reality.

Having that clear picture in my head as if I were really achieving it and living it at that very moment kept me motivated day after day and year after year. That same philosophy and approach inspires me today. In fact, I pictured this book on shelves a year before I even started writing it. As I got closer and closer to becoming a published author, I could clearly see my book on shelves, see myself in front of audiences on book tours, and see myself being successful while impacting many. I see outcomes of ambitions before they happen, feel what it is like to experience their success, and then I make dreams happen. I use that strategy for everything that is meaningful to me, and I've seen it work incredibly well time and time again. It's not a form of spiritual manifestation or anything like that. It is basically having a clear goal in mind that is so vivid you can feel it like it is real; therefore, apply yourself and make it real. I also used the influence of role models who have accomplished great things in their lives and thought of them as I would train and prepare myself for my future success. I would literally say in my head, "What would Pre do?" Or I would focus on a specific bodybuilder like my top bodybuilding role models Jay Cutler and Troy Alves and imagine what they would do in my situation. Quitting was never an option; success became the only option.

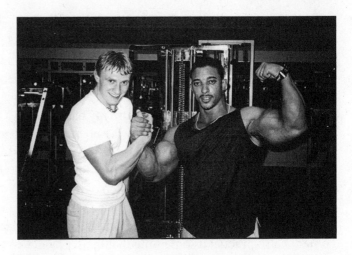

*Robert with first
personal trainer
Troy Alves –
Phoenix, AZ 2001*

My advice for you is to make a list of the things you like, love, and are passionate about. Put them in their own lists to clearly identify your priorities.

For me, a short list to show an example may look like this:

Things in life that I:

Like	**Love**	**Passionate About**
Playing basketball	Doing my own thing	Writing
Traveling	My family	Being the best
Spending time with friends	Animals	Being successful
Eating	Exercising	Changing lives
Working hard	Accomplishing goals	Being a role model

From that short list you can see some of my interests and where they rank in priority. There are some activities that I clearly like, others that I claim to love, and others that make me at my very best. If from that list, writing, being the best, being successful, changing lives, and being a role model are the things I am most passionate about, it seems fitting that writing books, going on tour, and being a positive role model is perfect for me, and that is what I do. You can also see that a very fun life for me would be spending time with friends, working hard, and playing basketball. But that would just be fun, not something that drives me in my life every day. You can see that I love to do my own thing, exercise, and accomplish goals. That is pretty good too, a fulfilling life for sure. But it is the list of passionate interests that really makes a person at his or her very best, and you can see that by reviewing my most cherished interests.

Make your own lists and be honest with yourself. List 5 to 10 interests for each category for a total of 15 to 30 so you have plenty of things to mix and match to create some career paths for yourself. Once you have made your lists of things you really, truly like, love, and are passionate about, then figure out a way to incorporate the things you love and are passionate about into your current life, and find ways to match them up with some career aspirations.

When you make it clear to yourself where your priorities lie, it is so much easier to map out a career plan and absolutely turn your passion into a career. It's so much easier than it appears. It is so fulfilling and rewarding you'll wish everyone close to you in your life understood how to make their own best life possible. You can share with them some strategies and techniques you take away from this book, and you'll have an incredible resource when my 300-page book *Take Action and Make it Happen—Bringing Out the Best in You* comes out in the future. I think it makes sense to learn from those who have accomplished what we're trying to accomplish because they can save us so much time, energy, heartache, and headache. Seek out experts, role models, and people who truly love their jobs and learn from them. Learn how they turned their passion into their career or how they learned to become passionate about their career. Living for seven out of seven days a week is something we all deserve and clearly something we should all strive to do. Life is too short to enjoy two-sevenths of it. Make your best life happen today.

Robert's Recap of ways to turn your passion into a career

We all have different standards and expectations for fulfillment. We have our own personal lives and our own unique interests. It is my desire that you really do find what you are passionate about and make a career out of it. We're all trying to win in this game of life. We're trying to win with success, win with fulfilling experiences, win with great lifestyle rewards, win with contribution and caring, and win with a love for life. I'd like to quote my hero Steve Prefontaine again, when referring to winning when he said, "I don't want to win unless I know I've done my best. And the only way I know to do that, is to run out front and flat out until I have nothing left." That statement resonates with me and hits home because I feel the same way about my daily experiences and about life in general. I have a hard time accepting something unless I have given it my best effort or unless I feel like I have earned it. It just means more to me to earn something rather than be given something. Some of us will take success any way we can whether we've earned it or not, but I challenge you to set a higher standard and work hard for your rewards. A strong work ethic helps out every area of life and will surely help you find passion and turn it into a rewarding career.

Robert's Top 10 tips to turn your passion into a career

1. Love what you're doing and spend a lot of time doing it. Spend the majority of your time doing your favorite things, and it will naturally turn what you love into more than just a hobby.

2. Believe in what you're doing and do so sincerely. When you display authenticity, you are perceived much differently than when you don't. Genuine people are often given more opportunities to turn their passion into a career because aspects like work ethic will never be in question.

3. Care more than others are willing to care and work harder than others are willing to work. This seems to always be a ticket to success in any area of interest.

4. Have a detailed vision for what you want to achieve so you have a road map to follow with steps all along the way that take you to your destination.

5. Develop the courage to follow dreams and pursue excellence even in the face of obstacles or adversity. There is nothing better than achieving dreams based on your real, true passions in life.

6. Surround yourself with positive and encouraging people. This alone makes turning your passion into a career so much more possible than it would be without the positive support network.

7. Find people who are living their true passions and learn from them. Apply learned information to your own life to do the same for yourself.

8. Understand that the people you spend the most time with are the people you will most likely resemble. You will develop character traits based on the traits of those you spend the most time around. Make wise choices when it comes to who you spend time with. This could be the difference between success and failure in very real and

tangible ways.

9. Create a timeline for success that keeps you driven every day to take steps toward achievement. Celebrate each milestone reached and set new goals constantly moving forward.

10. Learn something valuable from every experience with failure and find ways to turn failure into success.

"Robert Cheeke is easily one of the biggest names in the vegan community, and with good reason. Robert has done so much building online communities to help vegans network with each other (including organizing an event called "Vegan Vacation" where members from VeganBodybuilding.com meet once a year) and taking part in festivals and events to raise awareness of animal cruelty and the benefits of a plant-based diet all across the United States. Having attended multiple presentations over the years that I've known him, Robert proves that veganism is a very positive way of life, making his message very encouraging for people to take control of their health to get the most that life can offer."

Edward Mason
VeganBodybuilding.com member, fitness enthusiast
The Woodlands, TX

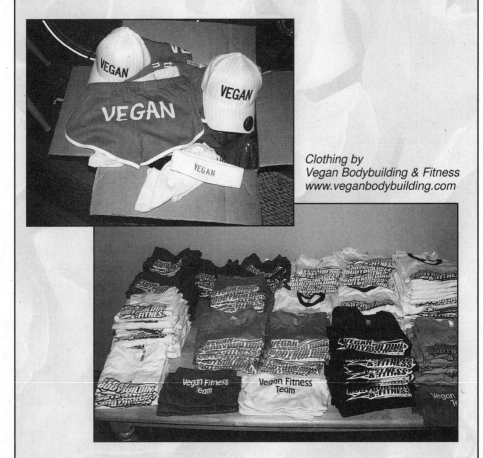

Clothing by
Vegan Bodybuilding & Fitness
www.veganbodybuilding.com

Chapter 12

Lists of Vegan Equipment, Products, Services, and Supplies for Bodybuilders

"If we are to fully embrace the vegan lifestyle and extend our compassion to the great lengths of our extended reach, we owe it to ourselves to be educated about what products have been tested on animals or contain animal by-products so we can make informed decisions and support our cause to its fullest."

Robert Cheeke, Author

People who follow a vegan lifestyle often focus on food as a primary objective, abstaining from the consumption of animal products through their food intake. However, there are many other areas of veganism to pay attention to including cosmetic products, clothing, and sports equipment. A football is often referred to as "pigskin" for a reason, and baseball equipment is often referred to as "leather" for the same reason. Clearly, a lot of our sports equipment from the balls we use to the gloves we wear is made from animals, and vegans need to know about alternatives. There are a lot of synthetic leather and rubber materials that take the place of leather balls, but since we're focusing around bodybuilding, I wanted to provide some insight on bodybuilding equipment that is often leather-based or containing animal products that can be found in vegan forms, including weight lifting gloves, belts, and tanning supplies.

Most gym equipment such as the pads on benches is non-leather synthetic material and most of the actual equipment inside a weight room or fitness facility is all vegan. The few things you may bump into that are made from leather are weight lifting belts, harnesses, and some padding depending the on the gym. It's the non-gym equipment that we use such as weight lifting gloves, belts, and shoes that are often made of leather. For those we have alternatives.

There are some great online stores and resources that have plenty of ve-gan-approved weight lifting equipment and supplies including: www.veganessentials.com and www.vegansportshop.co.uk. When it comes to vegan supplements, your best bets are www.veganessentials.com, www.foodfightgrocery.com, and www.veganproteins.com. All stores men-tioned are owned and operated by very good friends of mine. If you're in the UK, www.vegansportshop.co.uk has some vegan supplements as well.

The following is a list of vegan-approved products and their website in-formation:

Weight lifting equipment and accessories

Gloves

NewGrip Non-leather weight lifting gloves
www.newgrip.com

Valeo Non-leather weight lifting gloves
http://www.vitadigest.com/
valeo.html?gclid=COjlsID7wZsCFRBbagodYFnx_w

I use both brands and enjoy both of them. There are other brands out there too and online searches will help you find more options.

Straps

APT Pro Gear non-leather lifting straps
http://www.prowriststraps.com/lifting_straps

Shoes

FogDog non-leather athletic shoes
www.fogdog.com

MacBeth Footwear non-leather athletic shoes
www.macbeth.com

Vegetarian Shoes non-leather athletic shoes
www.vegetarian-shoes.co.uk

There are also plenty of non-leather athletic shoes made by New Balance, Saucony, Asics, Adidas, Brooks, Converse, Mizuno, and many others. Nearly every shoe company has non-leather athletic shoes and some have weight-training specific shoes that are non-leather as well. I personally wear New Balance and Saucony most often. There are lots of other vegan shoes for other non-athletic uses such as dress shoes, casual wear, boots, etc. and those can be found all over the Internet on dozens of vegan shoe websites.

Tanning products

ProTan – No animal products, no animal testing
www.protanusa.com

There are lots of vegan tanning products, but when it comes to bodybuilding competition color, ProTan is the only all vegan tanning product I know about for bodybuilding. I am open to learning about more and hope that there are more bodybuilding-specific vegan tanning products available. Dream Tan contains beeswax as its only non-vegan ingredient.

Supplements

According to Bodybuilding.com, the largest seller of supplements in the world, the most popular bodybuilding supplements are:

- Protein
- Creatine
- Glutamine
- Multi-Vitamin
- Natural Test Booster
- HMB
- Growth Hormone
- NO (Nitric Oxide)
- Anti-Estrogens
- Protein Bars
- Amino Acids
- Methoxy, Ecdy
- ZMA

These can be found in vegan forms and many of these vegan options and brands are listed in the Supplementation chapter.

In general, the best resources for your vegan supplements online are veganessentials.com and veganproteins.com. The owners of both vegan companies pride themselves on outstanding customer service and both ship worldwide. Both owners are also vegan athletes, incredibly outgoing and friendly individuals, and some of the greatest supporters of my company Vegan Bodybuilding & Fitness. I'm very pleased to call both owners my very good friends too. They are also two of the strongest athletes on veganbodybuilding.com (Giacomo Marchese from veganproteins.com and Ryan Wilson from veganessentials.com).

You can also find nearly every supplement you are looking for at your local Whole Foods Market or other good-sized health food or natural food store. Many popular vitamin and supplement chain stores have lots of these products as well since most of them, such as the amino acids, are vegan naturally. When it comes to protein powders and bars you'll want to make sure they are free of animal products. Every supplement, vitamin, health, or nutrition store will have plenty of vegan versions of these products made from hemp, pea, rice, soy, and other non-animal proteins. In fact vegan bars dominate the shelves in any health food store which is very inspiring and encouraging and powders are following that lead as animal product-free powders take up just as much shelf space as whey-based powders in many stores. When it comes to a few certain bodybuilding-specific supplements, Whole Foods Market and other natural foods stores likely won't have them, but stores like GNC and Bodybuilding.com will.

Below is an excellent resource list of vegan products found at http://www.vegforlife.org/athletes.htm:

Sports Accessories/Equipment

LEATHER ALTERNATIVES FROM VEGAN COMPANIES:

Cynthia King Dancewww.cynthiakingdance.com
Vegan Ballet Slippers

Heartland Products, LTD
www.trvnet.net/~hrtlndp/
Vegan Baseball Gloves

Vegan Wares
www.veganwares.com
Vegan Jazz Shoes & Ballet Slippers

LEATHER ALTERNATIVES FROM NON-VEGAN COMPANIES:

Adidas
www.adidas.com
Non-leather Athletic Shoes & Accessories

Asics
www.asicstiger.com
Non-leather Athletic Shoes & Accessories

Burton Snowboards
www.burton.com
Non-leather Snowboarding Boots

Circa
www.circafootwear.com
Non-leather Skateboarding Shoes

Evolve
www.evolvesports.com
Non-leather Rock-climbing Shoes

Fila
www.fila.com
Non-leather Athletic Shoes

Five Ten
www.fiveten.com
Non-leather Rock-Climbing Shoes

Fogdog Sports
www.fogdog.com
Non-leather Athletic Shoes & Basketballs

L.L. Bean
www.llbean.com
Non-leather Ice and Hockey Skates

New Balance
www.newbalance.com
Non-leather Athletic Shoes

Northwave
www.northwave.it
Non-leather Cycling Shoes

Spalding Sports
www.spalding.com
Non-leather Basketballs, Footballs, Soccer Balls, Softballs &
Volleyballs

Wilson Sporting Goods Company
www.wilsonsports.com
Assorted Non-leather Balls

* NOT <u>ALL</u> PRODUCTS AVAILABLE FROM THE COMPANIES
ABOVE ARE CERTIFIED VEGAN, BUT ALL COMPANIES
LISTED HAVE A VARIETY OF VEGAN OPTIONS; PLEASE
CAREFULLY CHECK PRODUCT INFORMATION BEFORE
MAKING A PURCHASE.

A general list of all vegan products for any need you could think of can be
found in a very complete and detailed list on:

http://www.peta.org/living/alt1.asp

A small sample from that website includes:

Ahimsa Footwear
1-877-834-3668 • www.ahimsafootwear.com
Vegan shoes, handbags, belts, wallets, messenger bags and
more.

All Vegan
619-299-4669 • info@allveganshopping.com
www.allveganshopping.com
Vegan shoes, belts, purses, and chocolates (available only in
San Diego).

Alternative Outfitters
626-396-4972 • CustomerCare@AlternativeOutfitters.com
www.AlternativeOutfitters.com
Non-leather women's shoes, handbags, wallets, belts,
watches, cell phone pouches, and other accessories.

Vegan Wares

011 44 12 7369 1913 • veganw@veganwares.com
www.veganwares.com
Non-leather shoes, boots, briefcases, wallets, dog collars,
jazz shoes, ballet slippers, and guitar straps.

Vegetarian Shoes

011 44 12 7369 1913 • information@vegetarian-shoes.co.uk
www.vegetarian-shoes.co.uk
Pleather jackets and belts and more than 50 styles of synthetic leather and synthetic suede shoes, including genuine
Doc Martens boots and shoes, Birkenstocks, dress shoes,
hiking boots, and work boots.

TheVegetarianSite.com

520-529-8691 • shopping@thevegetariansite.com
www.thevegetariansite.com
Vegan shoes, bags, wallets, and accessories.

Veggies Footwear

info@veggiesfootwear.com • www.veggiesfootwear.com
Vegan shoes for women, men and children.

There are phenomenal resources online and all it takes is some online searches like I did to find long lists of great companies to support and great products to support that allow you to participate in the sports you want to without having to use animal products and compromise ethics.

There are additional bodybuilding and fitness-related products that are vegan such as massage oils, sports creams, jells, and clothing. They can be found via online searches or using the links listed above.

Search websites such as www.veganessentials.com and www.vegansportshop.co.uk for a few more unique and specialty products commonly used by weight lifters. Use those websites as well as www.veganbodybuilding.com to keep updated as they get new products in stock, especially related to your vegan bodybuilding needs.

My friends who own HELD Vegan Belts not only make casual and functional everyday belts but can make specialty-requested products in-house such as non-leather weight lifting belts, wristbands, etc. They are located in Portland, OR and you can contact them via their website: www.m3house.org.

Robert's Recap of vegan equipment, products, services, and supplies for bodybuilders

The great thing about the growth of the vegan movement is that not only are vegan options popping up more and more at restaurants all around the world, but also there are more and more non-food related vegan options available globally. This is often seen the most in footwear. Nearly every shoe company in the world has non-leather shoes and has them clearly marked as such. This makes shopping for vegan athletic shoes, clothing, and accessories easier than it has ever been!

Online websites such as the ones listed in this chapter are often your best bet to find what you're looking for. Many of these websites are run by vegan companies who dedicate their professional lives to providing vegan equipment and accessories for consumers. They are worth supporting. You can also walk into any mainstream sports store and find vegan athletic tapes, straps, wraps, shoes, and other equipment on the shelves anywhere in America.

Search online to support the all vegan stores dedicating their lives to the vegan cause and also support your local retailers that offer vegan supplies in their stores in your region. Internet forums such as the vegan athlete forum on www.veganbodybuilding.com or www.veganfitness.net will have discussion boards about these topics so you can get product reviews, get tips, and learn from others who are using the equipment or accessories you are thinking about purchasing.

Robert's Top 10 tips for vegan equipment, products, services, and supplies for bodybuilders

1. Make an effort to search for the things you are looking for. Often the answer is right in front of you.

2. Read reviews of products or ask questions before you make purchases to make sure you are getting what you want.

3. Support all-vegan stores like www.veganessentials.com, www.veganproteins.com, www.vegansportshop.co.uk, www.foodfightgrocery.com, and www.cosmosveganshoppe.com as often as possible and encourage mainstream stores to carry more vegan items.

4. Join vegan athletic websites and participate in online forum communities to help promote vegan products you really like and to learn more about what is available.

5. Don't assume there isn't a vegan alternative for what you are looking for and settle for using what everyone else does. Do some research and come to accurate conclusions about what is available.

6. When there are vegan alternatives to non-vegan common items such as shoes or clothing, tell friends and others so they learn about what is available to them without causing harm to animals. Often times, people just aren't aware of the fact that there are animal products in their shoes, clothing, or accessories; if informed, they will likely make more compassionate decisions in their future purchases.

7. Thank the all-vegan companies for the work that they do to formulate, manufacture, and produce the products that we get to use to continue our athletic efforts using all vegan equipment, products, and services.

8. When you learn about a new vegan product that would benefit vegans and athletes to know about, tell someone like me who has access to a lot of people to spread the word to the masses. Share it publicly on your social networking websites too.

9. Make it a point to let your fellow athletes know that your training shoes, lifting gloves, or lifting belts are vegan. Many athletes may not even know non-leather versions are available and would be open to supporting a vegan weight-lifting product or accessory knowing that they are out there.

10. Train hard and make an attempt to represent a vegan product line or multiple lines like I do as an ambassador for NewGrip non-leather lifting gloves, HELD vegan belts, and Vega, a brand of plant-based whole food health products. Stand up for something and make a difference based on what you choose to support and choose not to support.

"Robert is a positive role model and champion, in mind, body, and spirit. His strength, determination, dedication, and sunny outlook fuel his success. I've had the pleasure of watching Robert manifest his vision from thoughts, to words, through to reality over the years. He's a powerful force on this planet, and I look forward to experiencing his continued growth and evolution."

Ani Phyo
Best-selling Author of Ani's Raw Food Kitchen
and Ani's Raw Food Desserts, *and Eco-Lifestylist*
www.aniphyo.com

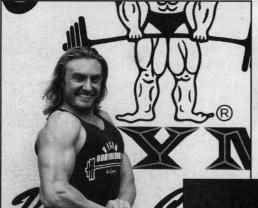

*Robert in front of the Mecca
– Gold's Gym – Venice, CA*

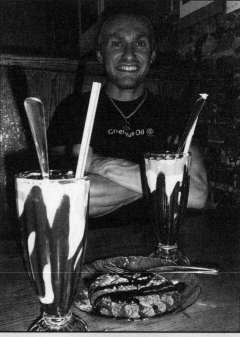

*Robert at the Chicago Diner –
Chicago, IL*

Chapter 13

Robert's Picks for the Best of Vegan Living in North America

"Nothing will benefit human health and increase chances for survival of life on earth as much as the evolution to a vegetarian diet."

Albert Einstein
Physicist, Person of the Century

I travel 30 weekends out of the year and have been all over North America. Because of my extensive travel, I figured it would be of great interest to an audience to learn which places around North America are my favorites for vegan living.

I have chosen a few different categories to highlight my personal interests and what I have experienced as the "Best of Vegan Living in North America."

My selections are based on my experiences throughout my life leading up to June, 2009. All of my choices are based on my opinions only, not surveys, hearsay, or any studies— just my personal favorites.

Best Places to Live as a Vegan Bodybuilder

1. Los Angeles, CA

Boasts and Highlights:
- Incredible sunny weather almost year-round
- Home to the most famous gym in the world - Gold's Gym Venice
- Has an atmosphere of drive and motivation among its citizens
- Best bodybuilding culture in the world
- Most vegan-friendly city in the world (tied with Portland, OR)

- Most bodybuilding celebrities in one city
- Most vegan celebrities in one city
- Best opportunity to make a career as a vegan bodybuilder
- In 2010, will be the official home of Vegan Bodybuilding & Fitness
- Hosts the National Animal Rights Conference
- Home to more bodybuilding competitions than nearly any other city

2. Portland, OR

Boasts and Highlights:

- Arguably the most vegan-friendly city in the world (tie with L.A. in my opinion)
- The most vegan athletes sharing the same gym (24 Hour Fitness Hollywood District)
- More www.veganbodybuilding.com members than any other city in North America
- One of the most livable cities in North America
- Most #1's for cities in America based on progressive ideas (#1 in recycling, #1 bike-friendly, #1 green living, etc.)
- The current home of Vegan Bodybuilding & Fitness
- Location of the Vegan Mini Mall (Sweet Pea Baking Company, Herbivore Clothing, Food Fight! Vegan Grocery, Scapegoat Tattoo)
- Home of the Let Live NW Animal Rights Conference

3. Seattle, WA

Boasts and Highlights:

- Perhaps the best vegan-friendly district in a city anywhere in North America (the University "U" District)
- Considered by many to be Portland's big sister. Similar to Portland in many ways, just bigger
- Home of Mighty O vegan donuts, Pizza Pi an all vegan pizzeria, and other popular vegan destinations
- One of the fittest cities in America (when it is sunny)
- Home of Seattle VegFest, one of the largest Vegetarian Festivals in the United States
- Home of Vegetarians of Washington, the largest vegetarian organization in the country

4. San Francisco, CA

Boasts and Highlights:

- The home of *VegNews Magazine*, the most popular vegan magazine in the world
- The #1 fittest city in America
- Home of Millennium, arguably the #1 vegan restaurant on the continent
- The headquarters of In Defense of Animals is nearby in Oakland
- Home of the annual World Vegetarian Day Festival
- More restaurants per capita than any city in America, many of them vegan-friendly

5. Orlando, FL

Boasts and Highlights:

- Incredible weather year-round, perhaps the best weather in the United States
- Home of one of the largest Vegetarian Festivals in the country, the Central Florida VegFest
- One of the best entertainment cities on the continent—fun around every corner
- Has some of the great gyms in the country including Gold's Gym in Sand Lake
- Home of Ethos Vegan Kitchen, my favorite vegan restaurant in the country
- One of the top ten biggest concentrations of veganbodybuilding.com members

6. Washington D.C.

Boasts and Highlights:

- More veganbodybuilding.com members than any other city aside from Portland, OR
- Home to more animal rights organizations than any city in North America
- Hosts the National Animal Rights Conference and other major animal rights events
- Great vegan food can be found all over the city including at Java Green
- Home of many successful vegan athletes including bodybuilders

7. Boston, MA

Boasts and Highlights

- Home of the longest running and 1st or 2nd largest (by overall attendance tied with Chicago) Vegetarian Festival in the United States, the Boston Vegetarian Food Festival (2nd or 3rd largest in North America)
- One of the most progressive cities in America
- One of the fittest cities in America
- Home of the Boston Vegan Association and many great vegan restaurants such as Peace O Pie Vegan Pizzeria

8. Victoria, BC

Boasts and Highlights:

- One of the most visually stunning cities in the world
- Fantastic spring and summer weather for outdoor sports
- A quaint city with lots of vegan food options
- Hosts a strong collection of Organic Athlete members (www.organicathlete.org)

9. Phoenix, AZ

Boasts and Highlights:

- A long-time popular destination for natural bodybuilding
- One of the largest cities in America with great food and great training facilities
- Home of many inspirational Pro Bodybuilders including Troy Alves
- Has Fitt Quest, an exceptional training center

10. Toronto, ON

Boasts and Highlights:

- Home of the largest Vegetarian Festival in North America – The Toronto Vegetarian Food Fair
- Canada's largest and most popular city
- Home of many vegan activists and annual vegan and health-related events
- A hot spot for Vega and supporters of plant-based nutrition

11. Salt Lake City, UT

Boasts and Highlights:

- Great city for vegan food for all types of tastes

- Great animal rights activist community, home of nearby Ching Farm Animal Sanctuary
- Excellent fitness community with unlimited outdoor sports
- Hosted the winter Olympic Games for good reason, claiming some of the best mountains in the country as its backyard

12. Vancouver, BC

Boasts and Highlights:

- Home of Sequel Naturals, the formulators of Vega, a top vegan nutrition product line
- Host of the annual Taste of Health vegetarian festival
- One of the fittest cities in North America with stunning Stanley Park and many nearby mountains and canyons perfect for a variety of sports interests

13. Eugene, OR

Boasts and Highlights:

- Home of the Pizza Research Institute, known for its vegan pizza such as the "3P" pizza (pesto, potato, and pear)
- Portland's little sister with lots of vegan food options and an excellent sports town
- Running capital of America and a good bodybuilding community too

14. Las Vegas, NV

Boasts and Highlights:

- Home of the annual Mr. and Ms. Olympia Bodybuilding competitions
- Home of some of the best gyms in the country including Gold's Gym
- Home of great vegan restaurants including Go Raw and the vegan-friendly India Oven

15. Chicago, IL

Boasts and Highlights

- Home to the Green Festival Chicago, one of largest and most progressive festivals in the United States, and the Chicago VeggieFest, an annual vegetarian festival that is 1st or 2nd largest in the United States based on attendance (tied with Boston)

-Home of the Chicago Diner – Meat-free since 1983

-Home of one of the top 20 gyms in the United States, Quads

Honorable Mentions:

San Diego, CA – Known for its incredible sunny weather

Bend, OR - Home of the Bill Pearl High Desert Classic and #1 adventure city in the US

Tampa, FL – Many vegan restaurants to choose from as well as nearby St. Petersburg, FL

Dallas, TX – A growing number of vegan restaurants and organizations in cattle country

Major cities likely to be found on other "Best" lists when referring to veganism, green living, or fitness are the following places I haven't been or haven't been lately:

- New York City, NY – Likely a top three on anyone else's vegan list
- Atlanta, GA – Often making news as an excellent vegan hub
- Austin, TX – The home of Whole Foods Market and known as "Mini-Portland, OR"
- Pittsburgh, PA – This city's name comes up often when referring to veganism. A large collection of veganbodybuilding.com members are also based in Pittsburgh
- Minneapolis, MN – It has been years since I passed through there, but I have heard it is another great city for veganism and fitness
- Cabo San Lucas, Mexico – Modern city with a variety of vegan options in grocery stores and restaurants
- Miami, FL – I haven't spent time there in about half a decade so I can't accurately write about the current vegan scene though it is always a big bodybuilding and fitness community

I've been pretty much everywhere else noteworthy as great places to live as a vegan bodybuilder. The truth is any place can be a great place to live as a vegan bodybuilder. Some cities just provide more opportunities, have better gyms, have a better atmosphere for success, are more progressive, host better events, have better weather, and cater to the vegan or bodybuilding lifestyle more than others.

Robert's Favorite Vegan/Vegan-friendly Restaurants in North America

You've read my favorite places in North America to live as a vegan body-builder and in fact, I have actually lived in many of those cities including Portland, Salt Lake City, and Phoenix. I plan to relocate to Los Angeles in early 2010. I have spent considerable amounts of time in every city listed, some that I visit four to five times a year or more such as Los Angeles, Orlando, Seattle, and Eugene. Others I visit two or three times a year including Washington D.C., Boston, Victoria, Vancouver, San Francisco, and Bend. There are many other destinations I visit that didn't make the list, though they are great cities such as Denver, CO; Concord, NH; Ashland, OR; Columbus, OH; and Gainesville, FL.

Of all these places I go on a regular basis, I imagine that many of you are curious as to which places have the best vegan restaurants. I don't always eat at vegan or vegetarian restaurants when I travel because I am a fan of ethnic foods and because of my close proximity to Whole Foods Market in nearly every city I visit. However, I have been to many vegan restaurants, likely more than most people will visit in their lifetime, so I will share some of my favorite vegan and vegan-friendly places around North America.

As always, the more I travel, the more I will learn and will update this list based on my experiences. As of June 2009, here are the best places on the continent to get vegan food.

1. Ethos Vegan Kitchen – Orlando, FL (All Vegan)

Boasts and Highlights:
- One of my favorite places from the moment I went there which continues to top my list
- Friendly staff, fans of Vegan Bodybuilding & Fitness
- Supportive of community events
- Tastiest vegan food I have had anywhere

Recommendations:
- What's the Dilly Philly? - Vegan Philly cheese steak sandwich (my favorite vegan entrée anywhere!)
- Vegan Pizza
- Mashed potatoes and almond gravy

Location and contact information:

1235 N Orange Ave Ste 101,
Orlando Florida (32804) (at Virginia Ave)
407-228-3898
www.ethosvegankitchen.com

2. The Blossoming Lotus – Portland, OR (All Vegan)

Boasts and Highlights:

- Uses only organic, fresh, and vegan ingredients
- Created by a vegan chef Mark Reinfeld and owned by long-time vegan and influential community member Bo Rinaldi
- Awarded Favorite Vegan Restaurant in Portland by Northwest VEG
- Big supporters of Vegan Bodybuilding & Fitness

Recommendations:

- Indian Bowl – the mango chutney sauce is delicious!
- Southwest Bowl – Avocado, beans, southwest sauce, yum!
- Anything with their homemade cashew cheese (my favorite 'cheese')
- Soft serve vegan ice cream

Location and contact information:

1713 NE 15th Ave
Portland, Oregon 97212
503-228-0048
www.blpdx.com

3. Real Food Daily – Santa Monica, CA (All Vegan)

Boasts and Highlights:

- Multiple locations in Southern California
- Large menu with lots of mixing and matching options
- A great spot for a business meeting, casual gathering, or dinner date
- A favorite spot for vegan celebrities in Hollywood

Recommendations:

- Entrees and specials
- Make your own entrees

Location and contact information:
514 Santa Monica Blvd
Santa Monica, CA 90401-2410
(310) 451-7544
www.realfood.com

4. Nicholas Middle Eastern Restaurant (Vegan-Friendly)

Boasts and Highlights:
- One of the most popular dining spots in Portland, OR
- Centrally located in the conversion of SW, NW, SE, and NE Portland
- Unfortunately closed by 9PM, so go early and expect to have to be on a waiting list for dinner. It is worth your wait.

Recommendations:
- Spinach Pie
- Vegan Mezza Platter

Location and contact information:
318 SE Grand Ave
Portland, OR 97214
(503) 235-5123
http://nicholasrestaurant.com

5. Wayward Café – Seattle, WA (All Vegan)

Boasts and Highlights:
- Phenomenal breakfast selection
- Large portions
- Very reasonable prices
- Excellent food

Recommendations:
- Breakfast any time of day

Location and contact information:
901 NE 55th St
Seattle, WA 98105
(206) 524-0204
www.**wayward**vegan**cafe**.com

6. Nearly Normals – Corvallis, OR (All Vegetarian and Vegan Friendly)

Boasts and Highlights:
- Oldest and best vegetarian restaurant in Corvallis
- Large quantities
- One of the best salads I've ever had and great vegan menu!

Recommendations:
- Sun burger
- Wild Iris Platter
- Smoothies
- Large Normal's Salad (my favorite salad anywhere!)

Location and contact information:
109 NW 15th Street
Corvallis, OR 99330
541.753.0791
www.nearlynormals.com

7. Green Café –Scottsdale, AZ (All Vegan)

Boasts and Highlights:
- Friendly staff that keeps the restaurant open later than scheduled hours when I show up with lots of friends
- Conveniently located on Scottsdale Rd.
- Amazing desserts!

Recommendations:
- Frozen ice cream-like desserts with fruit
- Most entrées are excellent

Location and contact information:
2240 N Scottsdale Rd # 8
Tempe, AZ 85281-1143
(480) 941-9003
www.greenvegetarian.com

8. Java Green Cafe – Washington, D.C. (All Vegan)

Boasts and Highlights:
- Extremely friendly and outgoing owner DJ Kim
- Great variety of fresh organic dishes

Recommendations:
- Just ask DJ, he is the man!

Location and contact information:
1020 19th Street N.W.
Washington *D.C.* 20036.
(202) 775-8899
www.javagreencafe.com

9. Proper Eats – Portland, OR (All Vegan)

Boasts and Highlights:
- Awesome owners Piper and James. They have supported Vegan Body-building & Fitness for years!
- Located in North Portland in a beautiful historic district
- Live music and political activism going on weekly

Recommendations:
- Tempeh Reuben Sandwich (my favorite sandwich anywhere!)
- Nachos
- Shop at their market too!

Location and contact information:
8638 N. Lombard Ave.
Portland, OR. 97203
(503) 445-2007
www.propereats.org

10. Hungry Tiger Too – Portland, OR (Vegan-Friendly)

Boasts and Highlights:
- Large vegan menu full of vegan comfort foods
- Large portions at affordable prices
- Vegans and non-vegans will enjoy the food equally based on variety

Recommendations:
- Tater tots
- Vegan corndogs
- Southeast vegan club sandwich (my 2nd favorite sandwich anywhere!)

Location and contact information:

207 SE 12th
Portland, OR 97214
(503) 238-4321
www.myspace.com/hungrytigertoo

11. Herbivore – San Francisco, CA (All Vegan)

Boasts and Highlights:

- They are good friends with Joe Connelly, Publisher of *VegNews Magazine*, so go with him and it will be an awesome experience.

Recommendations:

- Get whatever Joe's getting or whatever he suggests. He's been there many times.

Location and contact information:

531 Divisadero St
San Francisco, CA 94117-2212
(415) 885-7133
www.herbivorerestaurant.com

12. Pizza Pi – Seattle, WA (All Vegan)

Boasts and Highlights:

- Big Fans of Vegan Bodybuilding and that is always appreciated!
- Awesome owners and great place to take vegan and non-vegan friends

Recommendations:

- PIZZA!
- MORE PIZZA!

Location and contact information:

5500 University Way NE
Seattle, WA 98105-3521
(206) 343-1415
www.pizza-pi.net

13. California Vegan – Los Angeles, CA (All Vegan)

Boasts and Highlights:
- Cool place to meet up with friends and bump into locals
- Convenient location on Santa Monica Blvd.

Recommendations:
- Ask the friendly staff.
- Thai Salad is great too!

Location and contact information:
12113 Santa Monica Blvd #207
Los Angeles, CA 90025
(310) 207-4798
www.californiavegan.com

14. Go Raw Cafe– Las Vegas, NV (All Vegan)

Boasts and Highlights:
- The BEST raw food entreés I've had!
- Located in Las Vegas and has two locations!

Recommendations:
- Ask the staff. I asked and loved what I got. I think they were raw vegan wraps, and they rocked.

Location and contact information:
2910 Lake East Dr
Las Vegas, NV 89117-2203
(702) 254-5382
www.store.gorawcafe.com

15. India Oven in Las Vegas, NV (Vegan-Friendly)

Boasts and Highlights:
- All you can eat buffet! I go to town and eat until I can't walk along the Las Vegas strip anymore and have to take a nap or lie down in my hotel room

Recommendations:
- Eat as much as you can. It's good food, and like many things in Vegas, it's worth the investment.

Location and contact information:

2218 Paradise Rd. (at Sahara)
Las Vegas NV 89104
(702) 366-0222
www.indiaovenlasvegas.com

Honorable Mentions:

Pizza Research Institute – Eugene, OR
Chaco Canyon – Seattle, WA
Green Cuisine - Victoria, BC
Laurelthirst Public House – Portland, OR
Red and Black Café – Portland, OR
Chicago Diner – Chicago, IL
Bye and Bye – Portland, OR
Veggie Garden – Orlando, FL
Vita Café – Portland, OR
Vertical Diner – Salt Lake City, UT
Peace O Pie – Boston, MA
Molé– Victoria, BC
Leaf Cuisine – Los Angeles, CA
Spiral Diner – Dallas, TX
My Vegan – Pasadena, CA

Look them up online. They are all great places. I find "Google" to be a good place to start.

Websites such as www.happycow.net and www.vegguide.com may be great resources in addition to general searches. The Internet is a powerful tool to find vegan food anywhere in the world.

Check out blogs and reviews about other restaurants since some of my recommendations are limited because I haven't spent time in New York, Atlanta, Austin, Pittsburgh, or a few other well known Veg-friendly cities yet.

My friend Yvonne Smith hosts a TV show called The Traveling Vegetarian at www.thetravelingvegetarian.tv. It is another resource to get feedback about vegan places around the world, including reviews in video format which are often helpful.

Robert's Recap of the Best of Vegan Living in North America

It is fairly evident that are there are some places in North America that are far better places to live than others if you're vegan. Some places have strong vegan communities, lots of vegan stores, a vast array of restaurants with vegan options on the menu, cities with animal rights organizations and networks, and obviously some cities are more livable than others for other reasons outside of veganism. Though I have traveled all over North America, there are a few key cities I haven't been to including New York, Atlanta, and Austin, but I've covered pretty much the rest of the continent, including over a dozen destinations in Mexico and many cities in Canada. From my observations there are some incredible places in this part of the world to live as a vegan, but from my experiences I have also concluded that it is exceptionally easy to be vegan anywhere, since all cities have grocery stores and markets.

Ultimately, you have to decide for yourself how important it is to have a vegan community and lots of vegan-friendly people and places where you live. I choose to live in cities based on the best environment for me to thrive as a vegan bodybuilder. That is why I have chosen to live in the most vegan-friendly cities in America: Portland, OR and Los Angeles, CA.

Vegan restaurants aren't boring or bland as some people may believe. Today, vegan restaurants thrive all across this continent and all over the world. There are amazingly delicious food options that vegans and non-vegans alike are sure to enjoy in restaurants all over North America. In general, the west coast of North America and the east coast of the United States seem to be the most vegan-friendly places anywhere in the world. People in the United Kingdom may have an argument there, but in North America it's all about the coast lines. That is where a lot of progressive people live and where a lot of progressive ideas are shared regularly.

My advice is to get out there, see the world, and see what the vegan lifestyle has to offer no matter where you are. It's a beautiful world that is waiting to be explored. Go experience it and tell some friends. Let's continue to spread this message and support those who are doing amazing things for the animals and the planet.

Robert's Top 10 tips for finding the best Vegan places in North America

1. Stick to the west coast of North America if you want to experience the BEST of vegan living including cities, restaurants, communities, and places of interest.

2. Visit popular websites such as www.happycow.net to find out what vegan places are available in the areas where you travel.

3. Support local farms and farmer's markets. There is nothing more local and nothing more vegan than local fruit, vegetables, nuts, grains, and seeds coming directly from the farmers in your community.

4. Read city, community, and restaurant reviews so you have an idea about what the communities or restaurants may be like, especially if you are introducing the vegan lifestyle to non-vegans for the first time. First impressions are quite important, especially when introducing vegan food to non-vegans.

5. Spend time in Los Angeles, CA; Portland, OR; Seattle WA; San Francisco, CA; New York, NY; Orlando, FL; Washington D.C.; Vancouver, B.C.; Toronto, ON; and Boston, MA and you'll be sure to fall in love with one of these great vegan-friendly big cities.

6. Visit Eugene, OR; Asheville, NC; St. Petersburg, FL; Victoria, B.C.; and the US Virgin Island, St. Thomas and you'll likely fall in love with one of these outstanding vegan-friendly smaller cities.

7. When you are looking to relocate to a new city, look into the vegan scene or community by searching for groups on social networking sites like www.meetup.com, www.facebook.com, www.myspace.com, www.care2.com, www.twitter.com, and other websites that focus on specific themes within their online communities. Learn about the cities to which you hope to travel or move, from the people who live there and are part of the community.

8. If you find yourself in anywhere America and are not able to find many or any vegan-friendly restaurants, know that most ethnic food including African, Asian, Indian, and Mexican food restaurants are known for their vegan options. Indian, Thai, Chinese, and Ethiopian are some of most common (and my favorite) cultural food destinations to have vegan-friendly food items based on my travel experiences.

9. Most health food stores such as Whole Foods Market have a plethora of vegan food options including salad bars, hot food bars, snacks, prepared food items, packaged foods, perishable food, and produce.

No matter where you are, you should be able to find a quality grocery store to locate vegan food. If you happen to be in a major city in the United States you'll likely find my health food store of choice which is Whole Foods Market.

10. Consider the non-food aspects of the vegan lifestyle when you decide where to travel or move as well. Is the city or town you're going to a hub for harmful industries? Is it politically in line with your values? Is the weather nice and the air clean? Are there opportunities for your career and other personal interests? There are always "non-vegan" aspects of life to consider when traveling or moving, so don't let veganism be the "end all-be all" aspect for you when you determine where to go.

"In late 2006 at the age of 19, I was diagnosed with an advanced liver disease that had gone undetected since birth. After hearing this news, I began my search for methods to help control my health. This is what ultimately led me to Robert Cheeke and his website. Following the vegan diet and an exercise program, I began to experience a greater ability to cope with my disease and increased health. I later met Robert in the summer of 2007; I found him to be an incredible source of inspiration for me and a great friend. Robert has and continues to enrich my life in numerous ways. As my health continues to improve today, I am thankfully reminded of the role that Robert had in making it happen. I continue to be inspired by his drive and passion daily."

Zack Johnston
Friend, VeganBodybuilding.com member
Tennessee

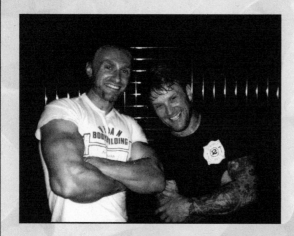

Robert with John Joseph, author and lead singer of the Cro-Mags

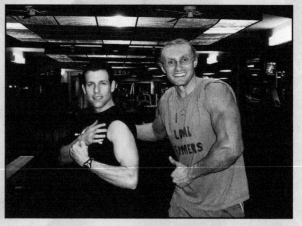

Robert with friend and fellow vegan athlete Javier de la Camara

Chapter 14

Testimonials from those who have been Inspired by Vegan Bodybuilding & Fitness

"My son got all shy when he met you (Robert Cheeke) and said, 'That's the guy on the DVD!'"

Steve Schimelpfenig
Animal Rights Activist
Vancouver, WA

"'Vegan' and 'Bodybuilding' are two words that seem to be completely contradictory, but Robert Cheeke has demonstrated that you can not only survive but also thrive as an athlete and bodybuilder on a 100% plant-based diet. I first discovered Robert as a result of my own journey to compete as an Ironman Triathlete and have high levels of overall energy and vitality throughout my busy life as a technology executive, without the use of animal products. I heard about Robert and ended up meeting him a few months later in Portland, OR. Since then, he has been an incredible mentor for me, both in terms of how to train effectively, eat effectively, and also as a shining example of how to set compelling goals and achieve them in the way that not only serves yourself, but inspires those around you as well. Robert's guidance has helped me to achieve a higher standard in my own life, and for that I am incredibly grateful."

Ravi Raman
Technology Executive, Yoga Instructor, Author
SetHigherStandards.com
Seattle, WA

"I've known Robert Cheeke for five years now and he never ceases to amaze me! Robert's energy, enthusiasm, and passion are contagious. He is an inspiration and a great role model for our industry. I am looking forward to reading all of Robert's books!"

Charles Chang
President, Sequel Naturals (Vega)
Vancouver, B.C. Canada

"I turned to veganbodybuilding.com when a former coach was giving me a difficult time about my vegan diet being inadequate for my training regimen. I knew from researching that this wasn't true and it definitely was not my reality. I was stronger, faster, and able to endure workouts that I wasn't able to complete before improving my diet through veganism. I recovered from my workouts faster and had a much greater energy source to pull from. I never felt better in my life; however, this constant nagging was putting a drag on my mental state. So I turned to Robert's Vegan Bodybuilding & Fitness website to see what other vegan athletes were doing regarding their training and diets to see if I really was doing it right. I got so much more than just that concrete information. I found a supportive community that I enjoy sharing my story with through my own training and diet blog. I love reading what others are doing and posting my comments on their blogs. This website has bodybuilders, power lifters, endurance athletes, martial artists, fitness enthusiasts, and cross-fitters just to name a few.

Robert strengthens veganism on an individual level. Just as a bodybuilder stacks weights on a bar, he is stacking up personal vegan success stories. Robert doesn't just lift weights; he lifts up the entire vegan athletic culture with his website as an inspirational resource. He presses viewers to reach their personal best in this positive community built around health and fitness. Robert fosters a society where support to reach goals is given, sharing of ideas enhances vegan culture, and networking of common interests is realized. Robert personally 'spots' this community to achieve more than they could have on their own.

Robert demonstrates real dedication to his cause and gives all of himself and his personal resources to it. He does not let fatigue or injury stop him as he is a true wellness warrior that does not quit in his battle. His belief that he can positively change the world leads him to do just that time and time again in true bodybuilder fashion. Rep after rep, set after set."

Mary Stella Stabinsky
Crossfit Trainer/ Veganbodybuilding.com member
Wilkes-Barre, PA

"Robert Cheeke is a vegan warrior. There are no other words to describe the man. He is a vegan warrior on a mission—one which he pours his heart and soul into everyday. From my perspective as a long-time vegan, Robert is definitely one of the most positive role models that I see in the world today. In my eyes, Robert is the embodiment of strong conviction, unshakable ethics, a 100% positive outlook on life, and a dedication to healthy living. After many years in the vegan community, I've seen plenty of people who would give veganism a bad name through

their poor diet and nutrition or negative and even destructive philosophies. Robert reminds us that (as vegans) it is our responsibility to live
our lives as a positive example of what a vegan truly is; what the vegan
world needs now is Robert Cheeke.

'Vegan Bodybuilding & Fitness' is the only book of its kind and is
an absolute necessity for generations of vegans to come. If nothing else,
Robert's book will help the many vegans who struggle with being underweight. I can say that because I would have killed (not literally) for
a book like this when I started my journey into veganism. At 5'10" and
115lbs, I had no idea that it was even possible for me to put on more
weight, get stronger, and feel more confident about myself on a vegan
diet. It wasn't until 2008 that I found Robert's website, Vegan Bodybuilding & Fitness (www.veganbodybuilding.com). On the homepage,
I caught a glimpse of the 2008 Muscle Contests and I said to myself,
'One day, I'm gonna be in those!' A year later, I finally started taking
my fitness seriously and I am involved in the Vegan Bodybuilding online
community. Through hard consistent training, a balanced vegan diet,
and the support and information I got from the Vegan Bodybuilding &
Fitness forum, I went from 115lbs and bench pressing 45lbs to weighing 135lbs and benching 100lbs in just 6 months! I also competed in the
2009 Muscle Contests!

I had the chance to sit down for lunch with Robert the other day at
one of Portland's many fine vegan restaurants and talked to him for a
couple of hours about the projects he was working on, his upcoming
competitions, and his plans for the future. I had always loved what
Robert was doing with Vegan Bodybuilding and Fitness, but after talking to him I found that he was someone I could truly believe in. He is a
guy who is down for the cause, who wants to help EVERYONE he
possibly can, and who will put all of himself into any challenge he takes
on. He seems like a guy who's capable of anything, and I after I said
goodbye to him that day, I felt like I could do anything too! That's what
makes Robert the perfect person to write the book (literally) on Vegan
Bodybuilding and Fitness."

Mike "Mikkei" Arnesen
Website Developer/Designer
Portland, OR

"I first heard about Robert through some vegan friends here in New
York City. As I learned more about what he does and who he is I knew
we needed to link our energies. As a full-time touring musician and
vegan triathlete with a background in boxing and martial arts I constantly get asked the same redundant question, 'You're a vegan; where
do you get your protein?' As a matter of fact when I had the great

privilege of meeting Robert at our show in Portland in 2009 someone asked me that exact question. You know what I did? I just grabbed Robert and said, 'This dude is vegan.' They were blown away. Honestly, I have to say, I was too. His P.M.A. (positive mental attitude) is contagious. I work with at-risk kids and recovering drug addicts to heal them with yoga, natural foods, and exercise. What I respect most about Robert is he's a doer not a talker. And if you just look at him you can see that. He's definitely someone who is going to have a huge impact on people, especially the youth because he's a shining example of what clean living and vegan bodybuilding can do for someone. This book is way overdue as he smashes the misconceptions that caring about animals, the environment and being vegan somehow makes you a wimp. I'm glad this compassionate warrior is stepping-up and coming to the mainstream as people like him can help save this planet by making proper food choices and building mind, <u>body,</u> and spirit. Right on Robert!"

John Joseph - Lead singer of the Cro-Mags
Author of *The Evolution of a Cro-Magnon* & *Meat is for Pussies*
New York City, NY

"The particular novelty of vegan bodybuilding is initially a pretty compelling idea for many people to come to terms with. The misinformation inherent in our common social scripts regarding how human muscle growth is fueled by animal protein consumption is deeply ingrained in our society. On first glance, the very concept of vegan bodybuilding seems a contradiction in terms to the uninformed. Robert has been able to use this seeming contradiction as a vehicle for reaching the hearts and intellects of people from wildly diverse cultural backgrounds and age groups.

When I asked Robert to speak at the high school for immigrant, refugee, and cultural minority students, he didn't hesitate to agree. On the day of his presentation, even though he was fighting that nasty flu of '08-'09, he didn't cancel. He got up there in front of the whole school, knowing he didn't look his best after not having trained for a while. Yet, almost as soon as he started speaking, the student body was enthralled with what he had to say. He dispelled some of the typical myths, and then he went on to inspire the students to follow their hearts. This wasn't the kind of meaningless, trite inspirational speech that so many people attempt to 'fix' young people with. This was a genuine recounting of Robert's experience as it related to him being the best he could be at his chosen goal against a significant pile of odds. Of course he was asked multiple times to flex, which he did with great joy and humor.

Another time, he spoke to a course I was teaching at the local community college. Again, he engaged the class with an informative and inspiring talk. It was bracketed by complex issues such as global food supply and activism. But the body of his talk was about how even though allowing one's inner drive to lead one into passionate work may not make earth shattering, historic changes, it will ultimately make the world a better place. This class contained a pretty varied representation of students. Robert made it fun and interesting for the whole group.

Vegan bodybuilding is becoming more popular and visible because of Robert. It's fair and correct to say that more people are living their lives in passionate and highly conscious ways because of Robert too."

Lisa George
Sociologist
Portland, OR

"Robert Cheeke is an inspiration to me, especially after beginning my own physique transformation. Plus I have had the good fortune to train with Robert on many occasions. And let me tell you, not only is the guy brimming with positive energy and enthusiasm, but he is absolutely ripped and chiseled to perfection. And believe me, when you're in the gym training with someone like that, it can be slightly intimidating. But this just goes to show the incredible potential available to anyone with an eye toward optimum physical fitness. And better yet, Robert personifies this without eating the flesh of animals, (since meat, dairy, eggs and whey are all fundamental ingredients of the bodybuilding world). Robert, on the other hand, illustrates how this can be done through a plant-based diet, which is much healthier for humans, animals, and our environment. So if I were to sum up Robert Cheeke in one sentence, I'd have to say he is a bodybuilder who represents, in every way, the greatest strength of all ... compassion."

Shaun Monson
Director – EARTHLINGS
www.earthlings.com
Los Angeles, CA

"Robert Cheeke is one heck of a vegan bodybuilder! I joined his website veganbodybuilding.com in late 2007. All I can say is wow! It totally changed my life. Robert was in fact the first vegan athlete I met through his remarkable online community. I have had the privilege of working with him at several different events that he attended in the Central Florida area. I could write many wonderful things about Robert, but then my testimonial would be the whole book. So I will narrow it down as best I can. First off, after getting to know the overall good character and depth of Robert, I can't imagine not having him in my life in some way. I've heard him speak on many different topics, including vegan nutrition, vegan fitness, and general motivation to get things accomplished. In all those talks I have carried away something newly learned. Robert's website veganbodybuilding.com is a prime example of the qualities and knowledge that he possesses.

I basically knew nothing about nutrition before I joined the wonderful mecca that is veganbodybuilding.com. Here, a variety of vegan athletes gather and share their knowledge, experiences, ups and downs, successes, and so much more. When you're around Robert or on veganbodybuilding.com you can't help but feel good and be positive.

Because this is all about vegan bodybuilding, of course the first place we met was at a gym! Robert is so full of energy at the gym that it's contagious. Seeing him lift heavy weights got me so motivated one time that I leg-pressed 400 pounds, which isn't bad for someone who isn't training to be a bodybuilder. Let me wrap this up by saying that Robert is an awesome human being, and the world better watch out because this vegan bodybuilder is taking action and making it happen!"

Hayley Suska
Friend, ISCA certified personal trainer, writer
Orlando, FL

"Had I never met Robert Cheeke, I would still be living an unhappy and unfulfilling life. Because of Robert, I have met the greatest people doing the most wonderful things, and I have transformed my life. Robert brings people together and is always more than happy to do so. His enthusiasm is plentiful, contagious, and always able to put a smile on my face. He truly practices what he preaches, and it has been a life-changing experience to be able to call him my friend."

Dani Taylor
Co-Owner, VeganProteins.com
Portland, OR

"Robert Cheeke helped me to see that vegan bodybuilding is not only possible, but that it can be done just as well as bodybuilding on an omnivorous diet. Before I found veganbodybuilding.com, I was working my way down from an obese weight and wanted to build a decent physique once I lost my weight. I became convinced by guys like Bill Pearl that it is possible to build muscle on a vegetarian diet. So, steeled by this information, I became an ethical vegetarian. I had pangs of guilt about still eating animal products, but was convinced that I would wither into nothing if I became vegan. Then I found Robert's website.

On the profiles section, I found pictures of Robert and Alexander Dargatz, two rather ripped individuals. I was shocked to see men with physiques like these on vegan diets. At this point, I had nothing holding me back from a vegan diet, and after reading a report by the UN on the wastage of animal agriculture, I had no choice but to go vegan.

I came to the forum section of Robert's website and found so much information and support there. Robert had some meal plans posted which I used to give myself an idea of what to eat when trying to build muscle on a vegan diet. The atmosphere there is generally very helpful, which I credit Robert for. He is a dynamic speaker, great motivator, positive person, and great human being.

If I hadn't come across Robert's website, I would probably still be a guilt-trodden vegetarian. He has helped many people attain a great vegan physique and make the transition into veganism. He is a great credit to the vegan movement."

Jacob Park
Writer, Personal Trainer
Chicago, IL

"Robert Cheeke is one impressive individual. When I came to www.veganbodybuilding.com I was shocked to see that there was an athlete who not only looked healthy on a 100% plant-based diet but also had huge muscles and a ripped physique. I wanted to pursue that healthy and strong image, so I joined his forum to find out all I could on how to be healthy and get stronger. I saw plenty of skeptics who tried to disprove what Robert accomplished with his physique. I don't think that ever stopped Robert, but it only fueled his energy to work harder in the gym and to speak louder.

Upon working with Robert at a major vegetarian festival, I saw how so many people were positively influenced by him. People could not wait to talk to him and take pictures with him. He pushes his positive image from state to state meeting people and letting them know that they can be fit and healthy eating a plant-based diet and doing exercise. I think Robert has a great aura that will dispel those myths about health and strength eating plant foods. He is definitely one of the most influential people in athletics that I have ever met."

Javier de la Camara
RAiN - RAW ALLIANCE (B-BOY CREW)
Former NBA Washington Wizards break dancer
Washington, DC

"Robert has been an awesome inspiration to me and many others involved in vegan bodybuilding and fitness. I first stumbled upon his website when I was starting my journey into really devoting my time to training hard in strength sports, as I was always looking for like-minded people who are vegan and share a passion for weight training. Ever since I first arrived at Vegan Bodybuilding & Fitness and began to learn about Robert and his accomplishments, I could see his dedication to the sport of bodybuilding and his passion for excellence in everything he does. Each year, he amazes me more and more, whether it be by stepping on stage to show off his hard work building his physique or through his many other projects. Robert never slows down, always keeping motivated to do more and more to spread the word of compassionate living as well as vegan bodybuilding. By example, his actions motivate me to follow in his footsteps and always seek to improve myself and the world around me; his positive attitude is definitely contagious!

Robert has proven time and time again that you can be successful in anything you put your mind to. As one of the most prominent figures in vegan bodybuilding, his experiences with diet, training, contest preparation, and other facets of the lifestyle make him a fantastic resource for beginners and experienced athletes alike. He's done great work to break down negative stereotypes by example. He has put vegan bodybuilding on the map. Whether you're just starting to want to change your lifestyle to be fitter and healthier or if you've been in the iron game a while and are looking for new perspectives to stay motivated and move your progress up another notch, Robert Cheeke is the person to help you at any level."

Ryan Wilson
Owner, Vegan Essentials
Waukesha, WI

"For you to fully grasp and believe what I am about to say, it would require you to stand before me and witness the passion and true feelings I have to say about Robert Cheeke. For now, I will try my best to express myself through writing....

Be thankful for the opportunity to get to know a man who works harder than anyone I have ever met. A man who has dedicated nearly all of his free time and money to support those he believes in. I just can't express enough how much he goes *above* and *beyond* with any task he is given; it's unbelievable! I have never had a conversation with him where he didn't say something positive or encouraging. He has taught me so much, and his personality has rubbed off on me. I can clearly see I work harder, volunteer more of my time, and am pursuing my passions more because of Robert Cheeke. Thank you!"

Stormy Given
Co-worker, friend
Eugene, OR

"The first time I ran into Robert's name was when I was turning vegetarian, then vegan, back in spring of 2005. At the time, I was working out consistently at the gym and didn't want to sacrifice my training to the diet change, so I started researching and reading a lot about the best way to combine the two in the most ideal way. And then Robert's veganbodybuilding.com website came up and I was astounded and overwhelmed by the extensive knowledge the website had to offer. I started to follow his regime and advice and saw the results coming. I was thankful that I found his website and articles. Then I kept following this phenomenon called 'Robert' since I realized there were more facets to him than just bodybuilding. He is about experiencing life to its fullest, every day, every moment, without letting any discouragement take him back. The more people underestimate him or his actions, the more motivated he gets. In some way, he reminds me of Lance Armstrong for his determination and focus on the goals he wants to achieve.

It was not until 2 1/2 years later that I met Robert at an event in Los Angeles, CA, and we got introduced through a mutual friend. Right on the spot we clicked and became great friends and have been ever since. In every visit Robert made to Southern California to stay with me while he was in town touring, he was fully charged and ready for the next challenge. While some of us have bad days once in a while, Robert seems to not have one ever, or at least doesn't show it to the surrounding world like most of us. He always has a plan from the get go in the morning, and no matter how the plan turns out, he knows how to make the most out of it and actually turns it into a better one than the original. And that, I think to me is the one thing I admire the most in him. It is always fun to hang out with him since he makes friends so quickly and easily even when different opinions are involved. When I need some lift-up and inspiration, I always call or email Robert and get that kind of 'injection' that gets me back on track.

What Robert has done to the vegan and healthy lifestyle community is beyond measure. It is a life-long crusade which still always feels like it has just started. I'm sure the whole world will take notice (and some already have) of Robert and what he is trying to accomplish.

Robert is all about a positive attitude and getting the most out of it, and I believe that if most people would act the same way, there would be a much better understanding between all human beings. Even when Robert is not into something he will give you the feeling that he respects it and thinks positively about it."

Eran Blecher
Friend
Israel

"Robert Cheeke has been an inspiring and heartfelt friend since connecting with him two years ago. From the moment I met him, I knew he was going to be one of the most influential people I'd ever get to meet. Because of Robert's website forum and his desire to bring people together, everything has changed for us. When I say us, I am referring to the devoted and loving relationship I am in with my partner whom I met directly as a result of a meet-up facilitated by Robert. We now own a sustainable business, VeganProteins.com, and I had the opportunity to compete on stage in bodybuilding side-by-side with Robert in 2009. Together we represented the vegan bodybuilding lifestyle and displayed a positive message of health, wellness, and fitness in a form of effective outreach promoting veganism."

Giacomo Marchese
Raw Vegan Bodybuilder
Co-Owner, VeganProteins.com
Portland, OR

"I always knew that living on a plant-based diet was the best way to truly optimise physical performance; but in the world we live in, we are often told otherwise.

It has taken the hard work of some truly outstanding individuals like Robert Cheeke to demonstrate to the world what many of us have known—that living a vegan lifestyle is a powerful way of attaining the highest level of physical performance whilst also making a positive difference to our world, humans and animals alike.

Even though I live on the other side of the world, I still find myself being inspired and motivated by Robert. His ability to bring the best out of everyone he speaks to is a true testament of his character.

His work in developing veganbodybuilding.com has given me an avenue to show the world that I too can become a great vegan athlete, and for that I am very grateful.

I look forward to reading many more of your future publications Robert!"

Joel Kirkilis
Vegan bodybuilder and Power lifter
Melbourne, Australia

"I have known Robert for many years, and I never fail to be inspired by his enthusiasm for the vegan lifestyle. I am a mother raising four vegan children, and although I am not an athlete, I do lead a very active life. I maintain great health and energy thanks to the obvious benefits of the vegan lifestyle. My children have also benefited tremendously from this lifestyle. They are fit, healthy, intelligent, never sick, etc.

I appreciate the fact that Robert has been an outstanding role model for fit vegan health. My kids have always looked up to him as inspiration along the way. They live in a very anti-vegan world, are surrounded constantly by neigh-sayers pushing meat and dairy at them (public school!), etc. To have the role model of an enthusiastic, fit vegan athlete constantly encouraging and inspiring is such a pleasure! Robert is always available to my family for suggestions, advice, and encouragement. He never ceases to amaze us with his energy and positive outlook. He is always available to my children, and that is a true blessing.

I cannot sing enough praises about Robert Cheeke. He stands out in the vegan community as a leader, yet he is approachable, friendly, and fun. I am excited to watch the strides he makes in his work in the vegan community. I enthusiastically support his work."

Leslie Otto Hill
Friend, Mother of 4, Whole Foods Market Team Member
West Linn, OR

"As a friend who has known Robert since elementary school, I can attest to Robert's consistent ability over the years to motivate and inspire others through his actions. He has been, and is still known for his legendary enthusiasm and his ability to set goals and achieve them—often with stunning success. As long as I have known him, he has always been an enthusiastic, energizing, and inspiring figure. Seeing Robert over the past ten years accomplish so much in terms of becoming a successful businessman and one of the most recognizable vegan icons on the planet has been remarkable.

One of his greatest achievements and examples of taking action and making it happen has been his ability to motivate others to make positive decisions regarding their health and well being. As a committed vegan, Robert has never been preachy but has taught and inspired others to alter dietary habits and rely less and less on animal products through example. He has also led countless others to create and maintain regular exercise routines. Moreover, Robert has been somewhat of an iconoclast by defying conventional wisdom and prevalent mythology regarding veganism. He has shown that vegans are not malnourished weaklings, but can be stronger and healthier than those that adhere to traditional American dietary patterns. Above all, Robert has been someone whose inspiration and actions will benefit others on multiple levels for decades to come."

Jordan Baskerville
Long-time friend, Robert's first training partner
Corvallis, OR

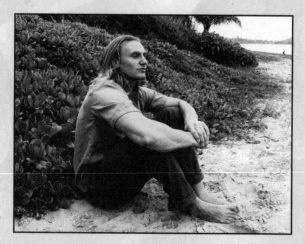

Robert on the
beach in Hawaii
(photo by Charles Chang)

Chapter 15

Final Thoughts from the Author

"The greatness of a nation and its moral progress can be judged by the way its animals are treated."

Mahatma Gandhi
Hindu pacifist, spiritual leader

I produce documentaries and interview people from famous bodybuilders to my roommates, and I always allow them at the end of the interview to add anything else that wasn't covered. My final question is almost always, "Is there anything else you would like to talk about that wasn't covered; do you have anything else to add about any subject?" I ask that question to give the person being interviewed a platform for free and creative speech to say anything they like and leave any final thoughts, words of wisdom, or points for the audience to contemplate. I am providing myself the same opportunity with this book since I'm the author and always have final thoughts to leave an audience.

Thank you reading my book. I do what I do for a bigger cause that is greater than all of us, and that is to reduce the suffering that animals go through on a daily basis. If I can have an impact on reducing suffering on a large scale, I am doing my job and will continue to work to do it better. It all started because of my desire to make a difference and because of my inherent commitment to work harder than most are willing to work in areas of deep meaning and personal interest. Building my body in the gym created every opportunity that followed. Vegan Bodybuilding & Fitness is the foundation of all my success and the base of my effective activism and outreach.

The very act of discovering what I was passionate about and working hard to achieve it, made me one of the most influential vegans on the planet. The same can be attained by anyone who believes in themselves and their ability to be great and do great things. Some of the most meaningful experiences of my life have resulted directly from my vegan bodybuilding lifestyle.

Many people have said their lives have been changed because of the influence I had on them. When people tell me they learned to believe in themselves as a result of my inspiration, I am humbled, honored, and thrilled to have played an important part in their lives. When I see animals living freely, being treated well, and saved from death, I am excited to see them get a fair shot at life. These are all enjoyable by-products of working hard to make a difference in the world.

I want to encourage you to do something outstanding with your life and to believe in yourself wholeheartedly and to really mean it. If I can go from a skinny farm boy to the world's most recognized vegan bodybuilder in just a few years without having any direction or understanding of how to do it but having the passion to pursue a lifelong dream, then I believe anyone can achieve outstanding results in their lives too. I am here to help; I am here to inspire; I am here to motivate; I am here to listen; I am here to ask questions and answer questions to the best of my ability based on my experiences. I am readily available and easy to find, and I look forward to helping bring out the best in you! And I am ready to be inspired by you too.

I challenge you to pursue something in your life that has deep meaning to you and that is something that will bring about happiness and fulfillment in your life. You need not worry if others support your ambition. I have made a living proving people wrong and standing up for something worth standing for. You can do the same; you should do the same, and doing so will be a very rewarding experience. Make the decision right now, before you put this book down, to do something exceptional in your life. Today is the day you take action and make it happen, and I'm here to support you.

I wish you all the best on your journey through personal growth to fulfillment and achievement. You can do it and you always knew it.

Thank you so much for reading my book.

With deepest sincerity and appreciation,

Robert Cheeke

APPENDIX

LISTS OF NUTRIENTS AND THE FOODS THAT CONTAIN THEM:

High-Protein Foods

Soybeans
Chick peas
Kidney beans
Adzuki beans
Other beans
Tofu
Lentils
Almonds
Other nuts and seeds
Kamut and spelt
Other whole grains

High-Calcium Foods

Black beans
Chick peas
Soybeans
Pinto beans
Tofu
Cashews
Almonds
Sesame seeds
Molasses
Dark leafy green vegetables
Brazil nuts
Hazelnuts (filberts)
Sunflower seeds
Globe artichokes

High-Magnesium Foods

Pumpkin and squash seeds
Bran
Almonds
Sesame seeds
Other nuts and seeds
Peanuts
Millet
Whole grains
Dried figs
Molasses
Black-eyed peas

High-Iron Foods

Dried fruit
Molasses
Chick peas
Black-eyed peas
Pinto beans
Whole grains
Sesame seeds
Other seeds
Prune juice
Dark leafy green vegetables
Jerusalem artichokes

High-Zinc Foods

Brazil nuts
Bran
Almonds
Walnuts
Lentils
Lima beans
Black-eyed peas
Other dried peas
Chick peas
Cashews
Pecans
Whole wheat flour
Corn and cornmeal
Spinach Asparagus

High-Iodine Foods

Seaweeds
Sea Kelp
Iodized sea salt
Dark leafy green vegetables

High-Mineral and Enzyme Foods

Miso
Vegetable juices
Barley green
Wheat grass
Papayas
Seaweeds
Citrus fruit
Tomato juice

High B-12 Foods

Wheat grass
Barley green
Spirulina
Cholorella
Blue-green algae
B-12 fortified foods like texturized vegetable protein (TVP)
Vitamin supplements

Vitamin D

Alfalfa
Chlorella
Blue-green algae
Fenugreek
Sunflower seeds
Coconut
Papaya
Rosehips

Essential Oils

Flax seed/flax seed oil
Olives
Olive oil

Other natural oils

Nuts and seeds
Vegetables
Avocados
Whole grains

Herbs

Parsley
Herb seasonings
Herb teas
Garlic
Onions

List courtesy of:

http://www.veganbodybuilding.com/?page=article_commonfoods

ROBERT'S COMPLETE LIST OF EXERCISES
FOR EACH MUSCLE GROUP:

Chest Exercises

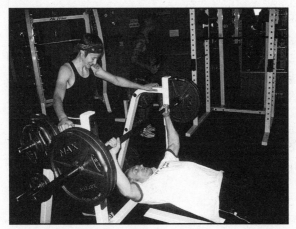

Robert training chest with Crystal Hammer spotting

Free Weight Exercises

- Flat Barbell Bench Press
- Incline Barbell Bench Press
- Decline Barbell Bench Press

- Flat Dumbbell Chest Press
- Incline Dumbbell Chest Press
- Decline Dumbbell Chest Press

- Flat Dumbbell Flys
- Incline Dumbbell Flys
- Decline Dumbbell Flys

- Weighted Dips

Machine Exercises

- Machine Chest Press
- Machine Incline Chest Press
- Machine Decline Chest Press
- Machine Pec Dec Flys (Arms at 90-degree angle)
- Machine Pec Dec Flys (Arms extended, slightly bent)
- Smith Machine Bench Press

Cable Exercises

- Flat Cable Flys
- Incline Cable Flys
- Decline Cable Flys
- Seated Cable Flys

- Standing Cable Cross Overs
- Incline Seated Cable Cross Overs
- Standing Cable Flys
- Standing High Pulley Cable Flys
- Standing Low Pulley Cable Flys

Bodyweight Exercises

- Push-ups
- Dips
- Plank static holds
- One Arm Push-ups

<u>Back Exercises</u>

Free Weight Exercises

- Dead lifts
- Barbell Bent-over Rows
- T-bar Rows
- Dumbbell Bent-over Rows
- One Arm Dumbbell Rows
- Stiff Leg Dead lifts
- Good Mornings
- Lying Overhead Extensions

Machine Exercises

- Lat Pull-downs
- Reverse-grip Pull-downs
- Narrow-grip Pull-downs
- Neutral Grip Pull-downs
- Machine High Rows
- Machine Low Rows
- Seated Machine Rows
- Assisted Pull-ups
- Back Extensions

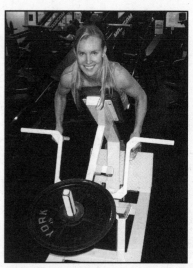

Julia training back with T-bar rows

Cable Exercises

- Seated Cable Rows
- Seated Angled Cable Rows
- Seated One arm Cable Rows
- Standing Cable Rows
- Standing Angled Cable Rows
- Standing One Arm Cable Rows
- Varied Grip and Varied Angled Cable Rows
- Straight Bar Pull Downs from High Pulley
- Cable Back Extensions

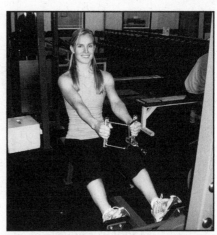

Julia performing seated cable rows

Bodyweight Exercises

- Chin-ups
- Pull-ups
- Static Holds on Pull-up Bar

Shoulder Exercises

Free Weight Exercises

- Overhead Barbell Press
- Standing Military Press
- Seated Military Press
- Clean and Press
- Clean and Jerk
- Standing Dumbbell Press
- Seated Dumbbell Press
- Barbell Shrugs
- Dumbbell Shrugs
- Dumbbell Lateral Raises

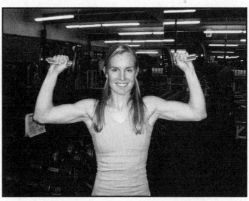

Julia performing overhead dumbbell press

- Dumbbell Front Raises
- Dumbbell Posterior Deltoid Raises
- Barbell Upright Rows
- Dumbbell Upright Rows
- Rack Pulls
- Power Snatch

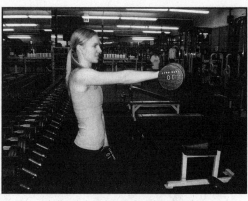

Julia doing front dumbbell raises

Machine Exercises

- Machine Overhead Press
- Smith Machine Shoulder Press
- Machine Shrugs
- Seated Machine Lateral Raises
- Standing Machine Press
- Seated Posterior Deltoid Flys
- Smith Machine Upright Rows
- Smith Machine Rack Pulls

Cable Exercises

- Cable Overhead Press
- Cable Lateral Raises
- Cable Front Raises
- Cable Posterior Deltoid Flys
- Cable Upright Rows

Bodyweight Exercises

- Push-ups
- Hand-stand Push-ups
- Wall push-ups
- Plank Static Holds

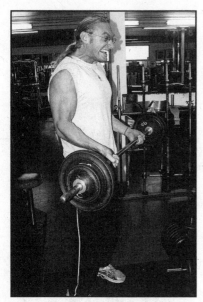

Robert training biceps
(photo by Giacomo Marchese)

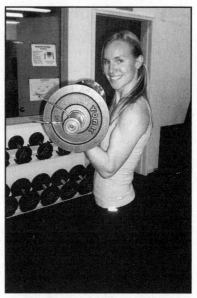

Julia doing bicep curls with the
EZ curl bar

Biceps Exercises

Free Weight Exercises
- Standing Barbell Biceps Curls
- Standing Alternating Dumbbell Biceps Curls
- Standing Dumbbell Hammer Curls
- Standing EZ Curl Bar Biceps Curls
- Standing Straight Bar Biceps Curls
- Standing EZ Curl Bar or Straight Bar Preacher Curls
- Standing Reverse Biceps Curls (pronated grip)
- Standing Neutral Grip Bar Hammer Curls
- Standing Barbell/EZ Curl Bar or Straight Bar Static Holds
- Seated Alternating Dumbbell Biceps Curls (seated at a 90 degree angled bench or slightly declined)
- Seated Alternated Dumbbell Hammer Curls
- Seated Barbell, EZ Curl Bar or Straight Bar Curls
- Seated Preacher Curls
- Seated Reverse Biceps Curls
- Seated Neutral Grip Bar Hammer Curls
- Seated Dumbbell Concentration Curls

Machine Exercises

- Machine Plate-Loaded Biceps Curls
- Seated Machine Biceps Curls
- Machine One Arm Biceps Curls

Cable Exercises

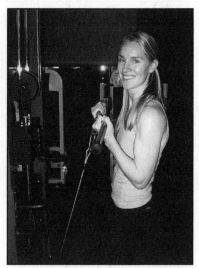

- High Pulley One Arm Cable Biceps Contractions
- Low Pulley One Arm Cable Curls
- Low Pulley Cable Curls with Straight Bar or Rope
- Cable Reverse Grip Biceps Curls
- Standing Alternating Cable Biceps Curls
- Seated Alternating Cable Biceps Curls
- Seated Cable Concentration Curls

Julia doing cable bicep curls

Bodyweight Exercises

- Chin-ups
- Pull-ups
- Static Holds on Chin-up Bar

Triceps Exercises

Free Weight Exercises

- Narrow-Grip Bench Press
- Skull Crushers (French Press) with French Press Bar, EZ Curl Bar or Straight Bar
- Dumbbell Overhead Extensions
- One Arm Overhead Extensions
- Dumbbell Kick-Backs
- Narrow-Grip EZ Curl Bar or Straight Bar Presses
- Weighted Dips

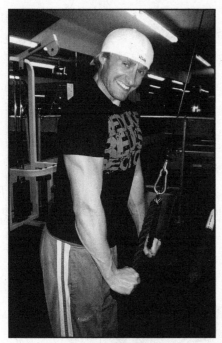

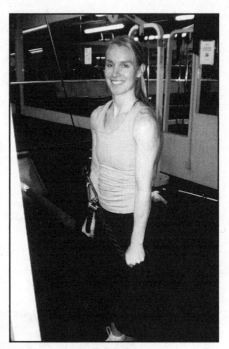

*Robert performing rope
triceps extensions*

*Julia performing rope
triceps extensions*

Machine Exercises

- Assisted Dips
- Machine Dips
- Machine Triceps Push-Downs
- Narrow Grip Machine Presses
- Smith Machine Narrow Grip Presses

Cable Exercises

- Rope Pull-Downs
- Straight Bar Press Downs
- One Arm Cable Triceps Extensions (supinated or pronated grip)
- Overhead Cable Triceps Extensions
- Overhead Rope Triceps Extensions
- Lying Cable Triceps Extensions (French press style)

Bodyweight Exercises

- Push-ups
- Narrow Hand Position Push-ups
- Dips using a bench or chairs

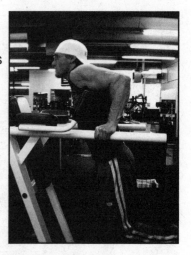

*Robert doing bodyweight dips
(photo by Julia Abbott)*

Leg Exercises

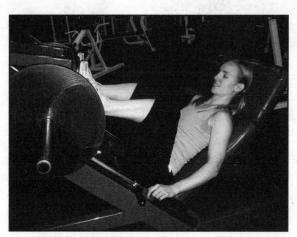

Julia doing leg presses on a hip sled machine

Over all Leg and Gluteal muscle exercises:

Free Weight Exercises

- Barbell Squats
- Front Barbell Squats
- Barbell Walking Lunges
- Dumbbell Walking Lunges
- One Legged Stepping Lunges
- One Legged Squats

- Dead lifts
- Power Cleans, Clean and Jerk, Clean and Press
- Power Snatch

Quadriceps-specific Machine Exercises

- Seated Leg Extensions (One leg at a time or two)
- Leg Presses
- Hack Squats
- Smith Machine Squats

Hamstrings-specific Machine Exercises

- Lying Hamstring Curls
- Seated Hamstring Curls
- Standing One Leg Hamstring Curls
- Smith Machine Lunges

Cable Exercises

- One Leg Hamstring Cable Curls
- Lying Hamstring Cable Curls
- Cable Leg Extensions

Calf Exercises

- Standing Calf Raises
- Seated Calf Raises
- Calf Presses using Leg Press Machine
- One Legged Calf Raises Standing on Ledge
- Donkey Calf Raises

Bodyweight leg exercises

- Squats
- Lunges
- Wall sits
- Box jumps
- Calf raises

<u>Abdominal Exercises</u>

Free Weight Exercises

- Decline sit-ups with Weights
- Side sit-ups with Weights
- Dumbbell Oblique Lunges

Machine Exercises

- Machine Crunches
- Machine Sit-ups
- Machine Twists

Cable Exercises

- Cable Crunches
- Cable Side Crunches
- Cable Cross Body Lunges
  (wood chopping (high pulley)
  lawn mow starting (low pulley))

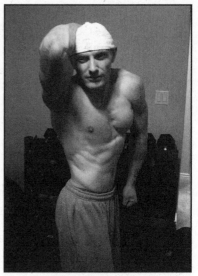

Robert flexing abs
(photo by George Wong)

Bodyweight Exercises

- Decline Sit-ups-Hanging Leg Raises
- Lying Leg Raises
- Partner Assisted Leg Raises (with resistance)
- Lying Sit-ups
- Lying Crunches
- Lying Side Crunches
- Plank Static Holds
- Yoga Poses
- Pilates Movements

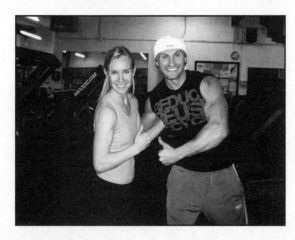

Julia and Robert after a
workout at Downing's Gym
(photo by Elizabeth England)

ROBERT'S RECIPES

Robert's Vegan Bodybuilding Trail Mix

½ cup Almonds
½ cup Walnuts
½ cup Pecans
½ cup Cashews

¼ cup Pumpkin Seeds
¼ cup Sesame Seeds
¼ cup Hemp seeds
¼ cup Sunflower seeds

½ cup dates
½ cup raisins

Mix into a bowl, serve and enjoy!

Robert's Vegan Weight Gainer

Mix into a powerful blender:

2 cups hemp milk
3 Tbsp organic peanut butter or organic almond butter
1 whole avocado
½ cup oats
15 grams pea protein
15 grams hemp protein
15 grams rice protein
2 Tbsp organic flax oil
½ Organic chocolate bar
5g BCAA's
10g L-Glutamine

Add ice and water as needed
Blend, serve, and enjoy!

Robert's Post-Workout Power Pudding

1 cup almond milk
1 cup dates
20 grams of pea protein powder
10 grams of rice protein powder
¼ cup hemp seeds
¼ cup chia seeds
Pinch of cinnamon

Add water or more almond milk as needed for consistency.
Blend, serve and enjoy!

RECOMMENDED READING:

Books:

Vegan Themed Books

The Animal Activist's Handbook – Maximizing Our Positive Impact in Today's World by Matt Ball and Bruce Freidrich

Thrive by Brendan Brazier

Thrive Fitness by Brendan Brazier

The China Study by T. Colin Campbell

Becoming Vegan by Brenda Davis and Vesanto Melina

The Engine 2 Diet by Rip Esselstyn

Skinny Bitch by Rory Freedman

Skinny Bastard by Rory Freedman

High Raw by Kevin Gianni

Striking at the Roots: A Practical Guide to Animal Activism by Mark Hawthorne

Meat is for Pussies by John Joseph

How it all Vegan by Sarah Kramer

Why We Love Dogs, Eat Pigs, and Wear Cows – An introduction to Carnism by Melanie Joy

Mad Cowboy by Howard Lyman

No More Bull by Howard Lyman

The Joy of Vegan Baking: The Compassionate Cooks' Traditional Treats and Sinful Sweets by Colleen Patrick-Goudreau

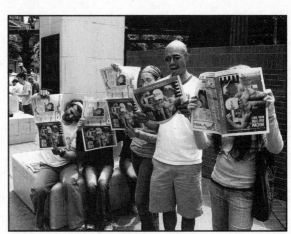

Robert's Front Page Feature in the Willamette Week Newspaper *being read by a collection of veganbodybuilding.com website members during Vegan Vacation 2008 – Visible members from left to right:* Giacomo Marchese, Dani Taylor, Jeremy Moore

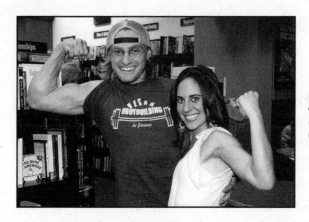

Robert with best-selling author of Skinny Bitch, *Rory Freedman*
(photo by Charley Korns)

The Vegan Table by Colleen Patrick-Goudreau
Ani's Raw Food Kitchen by Ani Phyo
Ani's Raw Food Desserts by Ani Phyo
World Vegan Fusion Cuisine by Mark Reinfeld and Bo Rinaldi
Diet For A New America by John Robbins
Food Revolution by John Robbins
The Kind Diet by Alicia Silverstone
The World Peace Diet by Will Tuttle

Robert's Favorite Books

How To Win Friends and Influence People by Dale Carnegie
Crush It! by Gary Vaynerchuk
Body-For-LIFE by Bill Phillips

Websites:

Bodybuilding and Fitness

www.veganbodybuilding.com
www.veganbodybuilding.org
www.veganfitness.net
www.organicathlete.org
www.brendanbrazier.com
www.veganbodybuildingbook.com
www.robertcheeke.com

www.veganfitnessteam.com
www.bodybuilding.com
www.veganpersonaltraining.com

Health and Wellness
www.renegadehealth.com
www.thekindlife.com
www.thrivein30.com
www.naturalnews.com

General Vegan
www.goveg.com
www.tryveg.com
www.thevegetariansite.com
www.supervegan.com

Animal Rights Organizations
Compassion Over Killing – www.cok.net
Vegan Outreach – www.veganoutreach.org
Mercy For Animals – www.mercyforanimals.org
In Defense of Animals – www.idausa.org
Farm Sanctuary – www.farmsantuary.org

Vegan Shopping
www.veganessentials.com
www.foodfightgrocery.com
www.cosmosveganshoppe.com
www.veganproteins.com
www.vegansportshop.co.uk
www.veganshorts.com
www.sequelnaturals.com
www.vegetukku.tarjoaa.fi/

Some of Robert's Favorite Websites

www.aniphyo.com

www.tonyakay.com

www.chrysander.com

www.godfist.com

www.thetravelingvegetarian.tv

www.garyvaynerchuk.com

www.gogladiatormedia.com

www.ted.com

www.vegnews.com

www.forksoverknives.com

www.organiclifestylemagazine.com

Blogs

www.lemonletter.blogspot.com – Wellness Blog by Julia Abbott, CPA and competitive vegan athlete

http://veganfarmgirl.blogspot.com/ - Vegan Farm Blog by Crystal Hammer, competitive vegan athlete and activist

www.sethigherstandards.com – Unconventional Methods for Outstanding Results by Ravi Raman – Vegan athlete, author and motivational teacher

http://girliegirlarmy.com/ - Glamazon Guide to Green Living by Chloé Jo

http://vegetariandeliciousness.blogspot.com/ - Vegan Deliciousness Blog by Carrie Tanasichuk – VeganBodybuilding.com member

www.ecovegangal.com – A blog by the environmentally-conscious vegan filmmaker Whitney Lauritsen

VEGAN BODYBUILDING FOOD GUIDE PYRAMID

Supplements
(powders, bars, vitamins,
minerals, amino acids)

Quality Fats
(avocado, hemp,
flax, coconut)

Quality Carbohydrates
(potatoes, yams, brown rice, oats)

High Protein Foods
(tofu, tempeh, seitain, nuts, beans, legumes)

Green Foods
(broccoli, kale, spinach, algae, seaweed)

Whole Foods
(fruits, vegetables, nuts, grains, seeds)

VEGAN BODYBUILDING TRAINING GUIDE PYRAMID

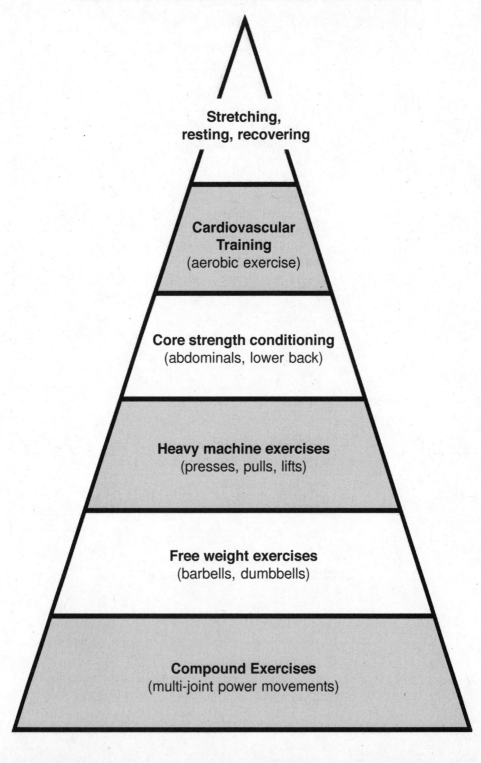

VEGAN BODYBUILDING LIFESTYLE GUIDE PYRAMID

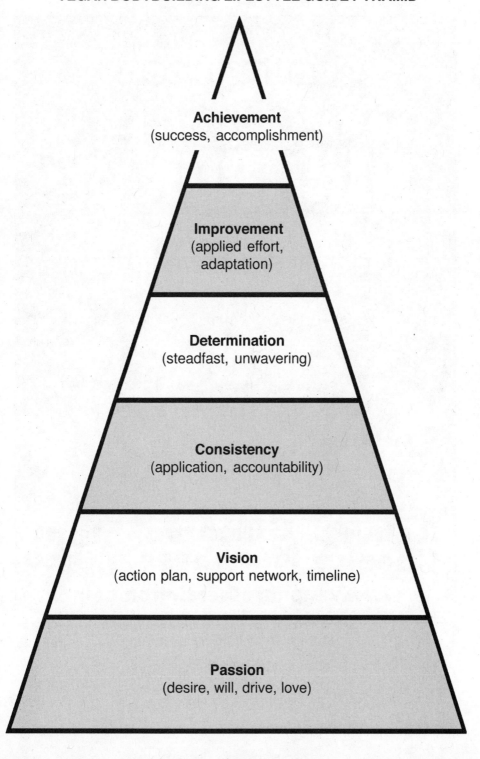

Achievement
(success, accomplishment)

Improvement
(applied effort,
adaptation)

Determination
(steadfast, unwavering)

Consistency
(application, accountability)

Vision
(action plan, support network, timeline)

Passion
(desire, will, drive, love)

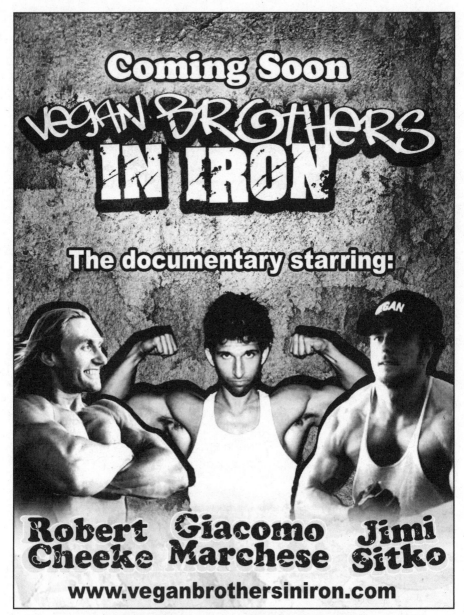

Vegan Brothers in Iron Documentary coming soon.
Graphics by Richard Watts – www.godfist.com

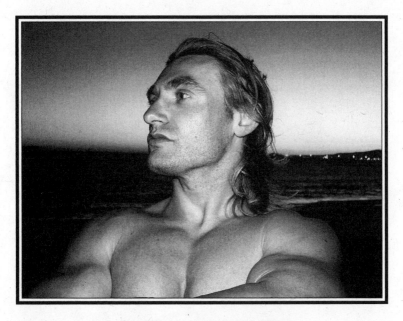

"Believe in yourself.
Whatever it is that you're passionate about,
resolve to make it happen today."

Robert Cheeke

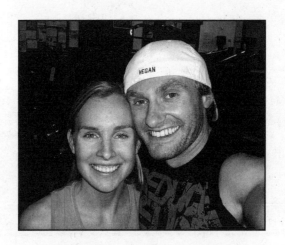

Thanks for reading!

– Julia and Robert